STRETCHING
THE QUICK & EASY WAY

STRETCHING
THE QUICK & EASY WAY

Dagmar Sternad &
Klaus Bozdech

Sterling Publishing Co., Inc.   New York

Translated by Elisabeth E. Reinersmann
Edited by Claire Wilson
Cover photos by Robert Srzentic
Interior photos by Robert Srzentic and Klaus Bozdech

Library of Congress Cataloging-in-Publication Data

Sternad, Dagmar.
   [Spass mit Stretching. English]
   Stretching : the quick and easy way / Dagmar Sternad & Klaus
Bozdech.
       p.   cm.
   Translation of: Spass mit Stretching.
   Includes index.
   ISBN 0-8069-8434-1
   1. Stretching exercises.   I. Bozdech, Klaus.   II. Title.
GV505.S7413   1991
613.7'1—dc20   91-13092
                                          CIP

10 9 8 7 6 5 4 3 2 1

Published 1991 by Sterling Publishing Company, Inc.
387 Park Avenue South, New York, N.Y. 10016
English translation © 1991 by Sterling Publishing Company, Inc.
Originally published as *Spass mit Stretching* © 1990 by
BLV Verlagsgesellschaft mbH, Munchen
Distributed in Canada by Sterling Publishing
% Canadian Manda Group, P.O. Box 920, Station U
Toronto Ontario, Canada M8Z 5P9
Distributed in Great Britain and Europe by Cassell PLC
Villiers House, 41/47 Strand, London WC2N 5JE
Distributed in Australia by Capricorn Ltd.
P.O. Box 665, Lane Cove, NSW 2066

Sterling ISBN 0-8069-8434-1

CONTENTS

For Whom Is the Book Meant?

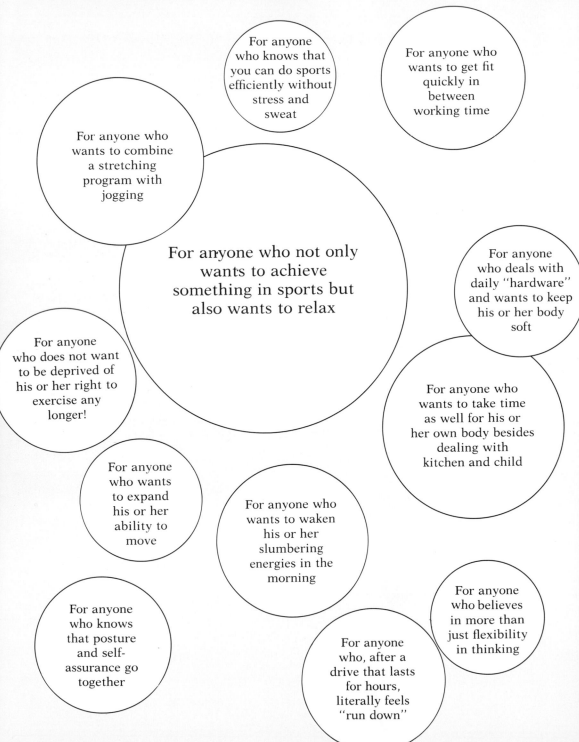

For anyone who knows that you can do sports efficiently without stress and sweat

For anyone who wants to get fit quickly in between working time

For anyone who wants to combine a stretching program with jogging

For anyone who not only wants to achieve something in sports but also wants to relax

For anyone who deals with daily "hardware" and wants to keep his or her body soft

For anyone who does not want to be deprived of his or her right to exercise any longer!

For anyone who wants to take time as well for his or her own body besides dealing with kitchen and child

For anyone who wants to expand his or her ability to move

For anyone who wants to waken his or her slumbering energies in the morning

For anyone who believes in more than just flexibility in thinking

For anyone who knows that posture and self-assurance go together

For anyone who, after a drive that lasts for hours, literally feels "run down"

WHAT DOES THIS BOOK OFFER?

The 3-Stars Program

- which you can start either as a beginner in sports or as an "old hand" in fitness matters
- which, with only 20 minutes daily, some inclination and the right mood will lead to increased flexibility, well-being, and enjoyment of life
- which, through its star and step concept, adapts to every standard of performance and progress
- which, with its exercise descriptions stresses the quality of execution for the exercises
- which you can do at any time and anywhere—at home, in a hotel, in the park, alone, in two's or in three's
- which, in all seriousness and with its scientific-based training background, does not leave out the fun of movement
- which is kept as uncomplicated as possible in order to save you from having to read yourself into the program unnecessarily

Four Extra Programs

- which make it easier for morning sulkers to get up
- which, with just a little more time, expand and vary the 3-Stars Program
- which offer supplementary exercises for the joggers among you
- which offer a freshing-up program that you can do quickly in the office in between work time
- which will awaken tired drivers

The Flexibility Test

- which takes situations out of "daily life" in order to test your flexibility in daily activities
- which measures the flexibility of the most important muscle groups
- with which you can find out where your weakness and your strengths lie
- which, with constant training, will afford you the experience of success

Additional Exercises for Breathing and Relaxing

- which are to be used as independent exercises, but also prepare you for and supplement your stretching program wonderfully
- which give you tips for deeper and freer breathing
- which teach you to direct your attention away from everyday routines and tensions onto your body

BEFORE IT STARTS

WHAT STRETCHING IS ALL ABOUT

Most of today's styles of bodybuilding and gymnastics emphasize perseverance and muscle strength. In order to achieve these goals, they require high strain on your body. For example, aerobics is a perseverance training that works towards raising the heart rate to 150 beats per minute, thus developing the endurance of the cardiovascular system. Bodybuilding improves the muscle strength and most of its exercises work muscles at 70 to 90 percent of their maximum strength.

Both are without doubt effective, but sweat-producing, methods. However, after an exhausting workday, not everybody has the strength to stress his/her body so intensively. The body often simply wants to rest. Here, stretching offers a gentle alternative: a relaxing workout that takes place at an easy pace and without stress but is also intensive and improves the flexibility.

> *Stretching is a gentle workout*
> *without performance pressure*

A new form of exercise, stretching combines active relaxation with systematic flexibility training. Stretching aims to improve the elasticity of muscles, sinews, and ligaments and the flexibility of the joints. The choice and combination of the exercises is made according to your functional-anatomical viewpoint. In addition, special emphasis is put on the technique of breathing and relaxing. That way, the effect on flexibility is supplemented and intensified and stretching becomes a comprehensive body training and provides a pleasant counterpoint to daily stress.

> *Systematic* ⟶ *Relaxation*
> *stretching of all*   *and*
> *muscle groups*   *Breathing*

Through deliberate breathing, relaxing, and stretching you will regain contact with your body. In other words:
- Stretching will put you in touch with the inner workings of your own body.
- Stretching will become an independent and comprehensive movement training as well as an irreplaceable part of a well-balanced training program.
- Stretching can be adapted to the needs of each individual. Because it is a gentle exercise method and does not require maximum stress in the areas of perseverance and strength, stretching can help you to stay flexible even when you are in your "golden years."

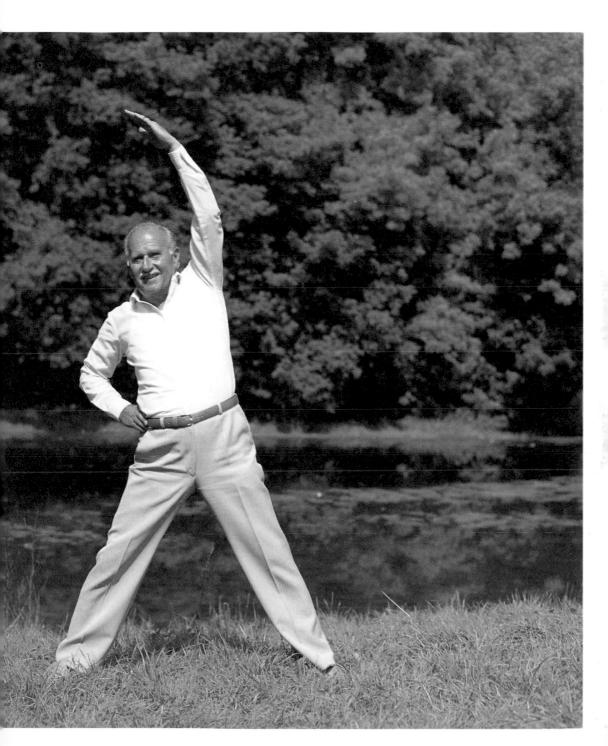

FLEXIBILITY—IMPORTANT FOR HEALTH

A pliant muscular system and flexibility of the joints are essential requirements for overall health and for the ability to perform everyday movements and sports activities safely and efficiently. Stiff or inflexible muscles and joints can impair your health in many ways. Too few or too restricted exercises cause tension in individual muscles or even whole muscle regions. A typical example of such tensions is the often clearly palpable "knots" in the shoulder and neck that can cause itching or stinging pains. These muscular cramps often become in turn the cause of headaches. If nothing is done to relieve such tension, which often appears totally imperceptibly, the muscles can become permanently shortened and lead to grave physical ailments. A common example of such atrophy is the shortening of hip-bending muscles. Through sitting too much, this strong muscle group shortens in the front portion of the hip. The result is a permanently forward-tilted pelvis, which then creates a hollow in the small of the back, causing pains in that region. By making counterbalanced stretches of the respective muscles, they can often soothe those pains amazingly fast. With chronic pains, though, you should always first see a doctor before you embark on an exercise program.

In the science of fitness, flexibility is equal in importance to the other components of performance, which are strength, perseverance, speed, and coordination. However, this fact is rarely recognized in sports and as a result, its necessity has been underestimated. Pushing yourself "to the limits" and sweating are still often considered the only measure of "effective" training.

Flexibility achieved through regular stretching is of great importance in sports because it greatly decreases the risk of injuries. Expandable muscles, ligaments, and sinews are much less prone to strains, tears and signs of overstressing when they are supple and in good condition. For example, it has been proven that the frequency of strains and lacerations in the upper thigh muscles of soccer players were lowered considerably through a systematic stretching program.

This alone should be reason enough to integrate stretching into each sports training program. But muscular suppleness also improves athletic performance by helping the athlete's technique to become rounder, more harmonious, and therefore more energy-saving. Last but not least, stretching is ideal for loosening hard and cramped muscles after an exhausting workout or starting a recuperation process.

All these reasons are valid for sports as well as for everyday movements throughout our lives. With increasing age our flexibility decreases. For many people it thus becomes also more difficult to carry out certain everyday activities or, for example, to face some dangerous situations safely. Stretching on a regular basis can help to stop or at least slow down this decrease in flexibility.

FROM STRESS TO STRETCHING

The key to correct stretching lies in a combination of relaxation, proper breathing, and concentration on your body.

Stretching relaxes

Does your everyday life include a lot of tension and stress? Do you rarely find time during the day to relax? Are you no longer capable of relaxing?

The relaxing techniques of stretching are an ideal way to bring calm to your body, mind, and soul. When practicing them slowly, they can help you center your concentration completely on yourself. In comparison to other passive-meditative relaxation techniques, the distinct feeling of stretching the individual muscles directs this concentration toward the feelings of the body and is therefore easily accessible to beginners. This way, your thoughts are diverted from everyday problems to your own body.

This mental relaxation in turn adds to the effects of stretching: If the muscle tension ("tonus") is high, then the limit of the stretch is low, but if tension is relaxed then the stretch limit can be increased.

Breathe deeper through stretching

Complete, deep breathing is imperative for the high-performance capability of the body. Flat and irregular breathing is an unmistakable sign of inner unrest and mental imbalance that will usually lead to psychic and muscular tension.

With stretching, you can learn to breathe more freely, and more refreshingly by developing the breathing muscles in the chest and at the shoulder girdle—a necessary condition for complete breathing. Calm breathing also increases the effects of the stretch. During the phases of inhaling and exhaling, the body undergoes a process of tension-building and relief of tension. By breathing deeply and consciously, you can influence your muscle tone.

Experience your body more intensely with stretching

In order to live in harmony with your own body, it is necessary to listen to its signals. In order to do that, you must first be able to perceive the signals—and it is exactly at this point that most problems begin. Many people are no longer capable of being conscious of their body, except when pains occur! Stretching is an ideal way to rediscover your own body and to enjoy its positive feelings. Through the stimulation of stretching, you can become attuned to the feelings of specific body parts, of the course of the muscles and of the margin of your joints. Through a stretching program that includes concentration on bodily feeling, the optimal stretching limit can be determined and, therefore, exactly the right stretching measure can be reached. This technique is totally in contrast to body building techniques. This process is discussed in greater depth and with more detail in the 3-Stars Program section of this book.

STRETCHING—
HOW AND WHY?

Stretching, as an exercise, refers to a specific body position that is held, without teetering, bouncing, or even forceful straining for a specific amount of time.

It has its basis in the effect of the so-called stretching reflex of the skeleto-muscular system. This reflex causes a muscle to contract as its fibres get increasingly longer, so counteracting the stretching. This is the cause behind the feeling of tension that we feel when we stretch. If stretching happens quickly, then the contraction will be earlier and stronger. As a result, the muscle cannot be stretched as far. Many exercise programs and sports nevertheless surpass this limit over and over again, resulting in muscle strains and at worst muscle tears. Painful or sore muscles that occur after doing sports are a sign of microscopic injuries of muscle fibres and tissue structures. The origin of sore muscles has not yet been definitely located, but it is clear that they are *not* a sign of good training!

Stretching works muscles slowly and carefully. It tries on the one hand to keep the stretching reflex as small as possible, and on the other hand to be kind to muscle tissue and the muscles as they are being stretched. Stretching allows you to expand and contract your muscles beyond their normal length, until limit is felt. This position is then held onto. At this point, the original feeling of tension, which should not be painful, should give way to a pleasant, warm feeling of stretching, and, as a result, the muscle can be stretched even fur-

ther. This change in the feeling of your muscles can be explained by a second reflex that comes into action, the so-called autogenous restraint.

If you practice stretching correctly, you can consciously experi-

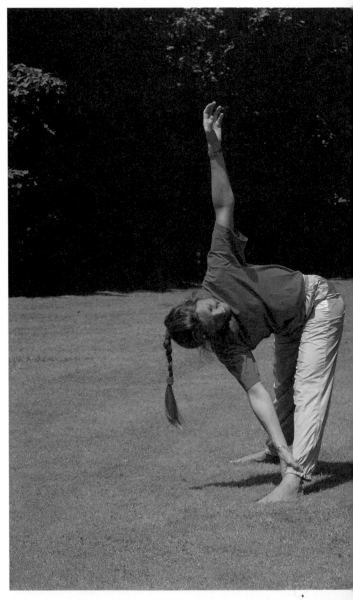

ence the processes of the stretching, tightening, and relaxing of your muscle fibres. For the beginner, such soft changes in the body are not always apparent, but during the course of the exercises they become the main experience of stretching.

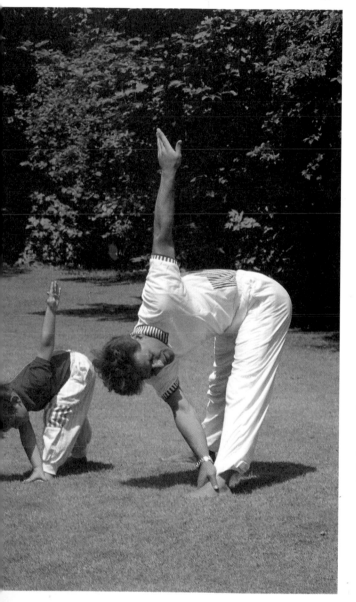

STEP BY STEP GUIDE TO STRETCHING

• Assume a particular stretching position slowly and carefully
• Stretch the particular muscle until you feel the barest hint of discomfort. Release the stretch as soon as you feel pain.
• Breathe deeply and continuously, while you hold the stretch, making sure to breathe deeply from your stomach (see "Breathing and Relaxing" on page 64).
• Try consciously to relax the stretched muscle or muscle group as well as your entire body during the exercise
• Hold the stretch for about 15 to 30 seconds, but don't count them tensely! The length of the stretch is based solely on your personal feelings.
• Direct your concentration alternately towards your breathing, your degree of relaxation, and the feeling in your muscular system.
• When the tension in your stretched muscle decreases, try to extend the stretch a bit and hold it again.
• Bring the stretch to an end slowly. The feeling in your muscular system should now become one of comfortable relaxation.
• Perform each stretch for a second time after a short break.

HOW TO BEGIN

When?

Before you begin, decide on the time of day that your new program will best fit into your daily routine. If possible, make time for it in the evening, because the muscles are softer and easier to stretch in the evening.

How long?

You should reserve at least 20 minutes for your new training. You need at least that much time in order to tune into the training session and to carry out a balanced combination of exercises. You would miss the point of stretching and its anticipated goal if you hastily did the 10-exercise session and just "wrote it off"! Be fair to yourself. Surely you can spare 20 minutes a day as a bare minimum to grant to yourself and your body!

How often?

It is best to perform your 20-minute-session daily. Stretching does not make you tired so there should be no problem with this regimen, even for beginners. With regular training, your flexibility will develop quickly and effectively.

Where?

Pick an "exercise corner" in which you feel really comfortable. It does not matter where it is—in the park, in the living room, in the office. The main thing is that you have this area all to yourself, because these 20 minutes should be reserved totally for your personal well-being— a time that you look forward to and that belongs just to you. The room, though, should be quite warm since cold temperatures increase the muscle-tension and decrease the stretching limit.

Music?

If you have the equipment, you can listen to soft music during stretching exercises. This can help to create a space around you in which everyday life-problems have no place.

But now it really starts—and do it with a flexibility test!

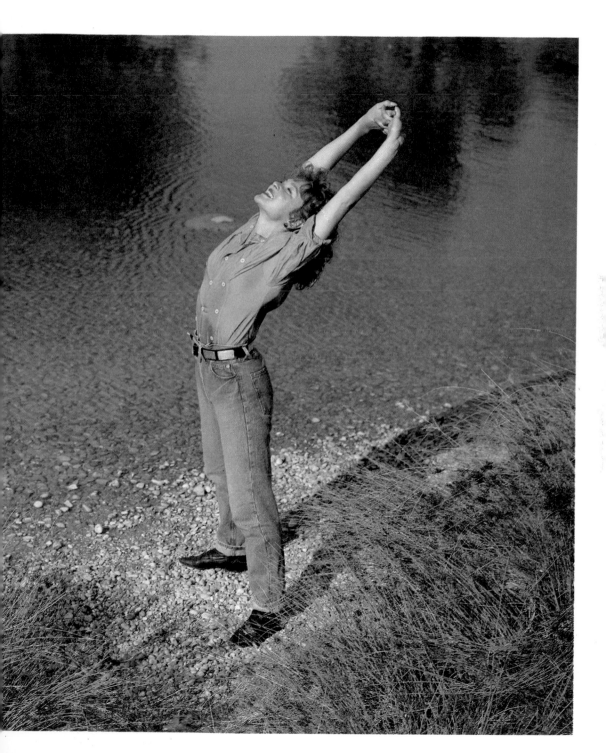

THE FLEXIBILITY TEST

How flexible are you?

Do you first have to sit down to tie your shoelaces?

Did you have problems the other day picking up a pencil that rolled under your chair?

When your back itches, do you have a hard time trying to scratch yourself?

The following test is aimed at determining the degree of flexibility/extensibility of your most important muscle groups. The subsequent five test exercises are based on everyday routine situations, because, after all, these are the situations for which you most want to become fit and flexible.

Should you warm up before the test?

Because the test aims to determine your everyday and hourly flexibility, you should take the test without any special preparations or warmups. The measure is not the splits or the upper-body bends that you can achieve after a comprehensive warm-up exercise, but the stretching that you engage in in everyday life. But this means that you have to be a little careful! Ambition and willpower are not appropriate: Only stretch as far as you can without great effort. An injury would be a bad start for your new stretching program.

Judging Your Flexibility

Practice all five test exercises in the order indicated. At the end of each exercise, you will find a small grading system that tells you if and how well you passed the respective test. If you have not yet passed one or more of the exercises, it is certainly not the end of the world. After all, you are a beginner and you are full of energy to overcome such small weaknesses. The test results are meant as an obtrusive but concrete indicator. Because once you have discovered your weak spots, then you can pay special attention to those exercises in the left column (Not Yet Achieved). Do those exercises in the 3-Stars Program not two but four times and also hold each of the stretches somewhat longer.

Regardless of your test results, there is no exaggerated ambition or even performance pressure required

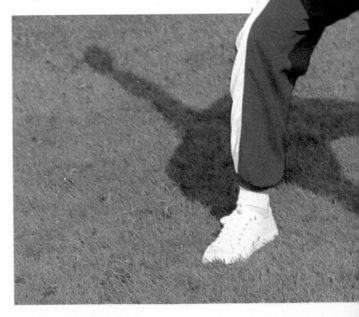

for this program! It is not a matter of achieving top performance, but of strengthening weaknesses and improving your all-around flexibility.

Passing the test—what happens next?

If, according to the grading system, you have merely "passed" the test, that does not mean that you can rest on your laurels. Your goal in the long run should be a "good" or even "very good" performance, as indicated in the two center columns. Even if you have difficulties at the beginning, these goals are by all means possible to achieve. You will be surprised about your ability to work up through the grades.

Everyday life is full of stretching exercises

In order to help achieve your goal faster, use every opportunity in everyday life to stretch yourself—instead of moaning that you dropped the pencil or spoon again, consider it a welcome chance to stretch yourself. It is a golden opportunity

—when the book you are looking for happens to be on the top shelf

—when you have to stand on the train or bus and hold onto the bar above your head

—when your child's toys roll underneath the bed

—when the windows have to be cleaned.

The test exercises are here merely to catch your interest, because everyday life is loaded with stretching exercises! From time to time, repeat the whole test, so that you can see your improvements. At the beginning you will improve very quickly—enjoy it! After the early rapid improvements, though, further progress will require greater patience and constant practice. Do not get discouraged—this is unfortunately quite natural.

1 THE SHOELACE TEST

You can determine how stiff or flexible you are when tying your shoelaces. The main focus of this exercise is increasing the flexibility of the rear leg muscles, which for many people are chronically shortened because of constantly sitting. When this is combined with weak stomach muscles, it may result in permanent deformation of the pelvis, resulting in chronic lower-back pain. This exercise will also help trained sportsmen, who often have problems with the flexibility of their legs, resulting from uneven stress on those muscle-groups.

Are you able to tie your shoelaces while keeping your legs stretched?

How to Do the Exercise

• In this exercise, as in all the following ones, very gently go into the stretch position pictured at right. You should not overexert yourself, and under no circumstances should you try to reach down with a swing. A muscle strain definitely would not be a good start.
• If you are actually wearing shoes with laces, untie and retie them. This way you'll realize if you are able to reach the tips of your toes with your hands for a long period of time without getting cramps.
• Keep your legs together. Are your knees still stretched?

Not Yet Achieved	Passed	Good	Very Good
Exercises 7 and 8 in the 3-Stars program cover this muscle region	You can tie your shoelace without problem	You can touch the floor with both hands	You can place both palms on the floor behind your heels

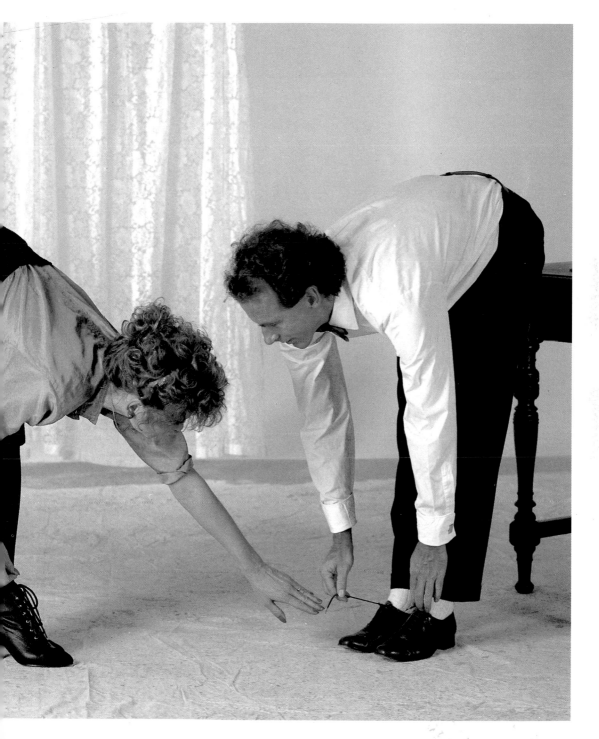

2 AN ITCHY BACK

Your back itches and you just can't reach it with your hands . . . you had problems getting into your jacket again? The flexibility of the chest and breathing muscles that determines whether you are able to scratch your back without problems or whether you can get into a somewhat tight jacket.

The test exercise for chest-muscle flexibility is certainly not easy. You will probably also have a "chocolate" side, and will therefore be able to do this exercise in only one direction at first. That is quite normal. Nevertheless, strive for a balanced and thus equal flexibility.

Are you able to bend your forearms, one from above and one from below, behind your back so that the tips of the fingers on each hand touch?

How To Do the Exercises

Some test runs are allowed, and your stretching partner may help you at the beginning.

Since the test exercise is somewhat difficult, this test, as an exception, is considered as passed when your fingertips touch on one side only. Nevertheless, the next goal will be to achieve this flexibility equally on both sides, since, after all, the system of chest and breathing muscles has to be expandable on both sides.

Not Yet Achieved	Passed	Good	Very Good
Exercise 2 in the 3-Stars program	The fingers of both hands touch on one side	The fingers of both hands touch on both sides	The fingers of both hands hook together on both sides

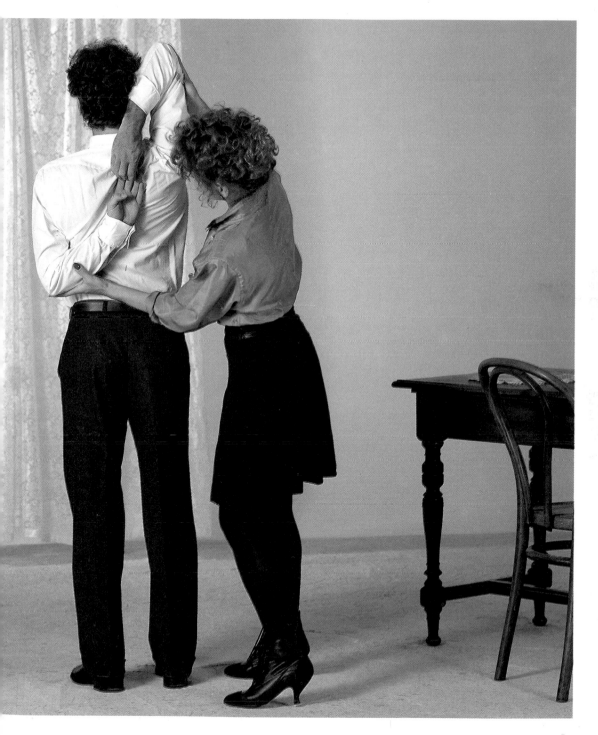

3 REACHING FOR THE FILES

Not very long ago, few offices were equipped with computers, swivel-chairs or other luxuries, so that a person was seated on a regular chair with four legs and the file cabinet was standing on the side or behind oneself. With this arrangement, one constantly had to turn around each time when one needed a file. The old-fashioned motions used in these activities were good exercise for the spine and the chest muscles. However, in our "luxurious" time, there is no longer any need for such motions, and a formerly routine movement has turned into an exercise.

While sitting, are you able to turn around in your chair so that you can place both hands on a table?

How To Do the Exercise

• Arrange a chair so that it faces away from the table. Sit down on the chair with you back straight, your soles flat on the floor, and both feet pressed against the inside of the chair legs.
• Turn around to the right until you are able to touch the table with both hands, as shown in the photograph. They should look like the hands on a clock at noon.
• Keep your back straight, and do not bend your upper body forward.
• Keep the soles of your feet flat on the floor.
• Do not slip on your chair—cheating is not allowed!

The test can only be counted as passed when you are able to turn your trunk in both directions. The Very Good performance does not necessarily have to be your first goal. How about halfway around?

Not Yet Achieved	Passed	Good	Very Good
Exercise 9 in the 3-Stars program covers this muscle region.	Both hands point behind the back—12 o'clock	Both hands point behind the back—1 o'clock when turning right, 11 o'clock when turning left	Both hands point behind the back—2 o'clock when turning right, 10 o'clock when turning left

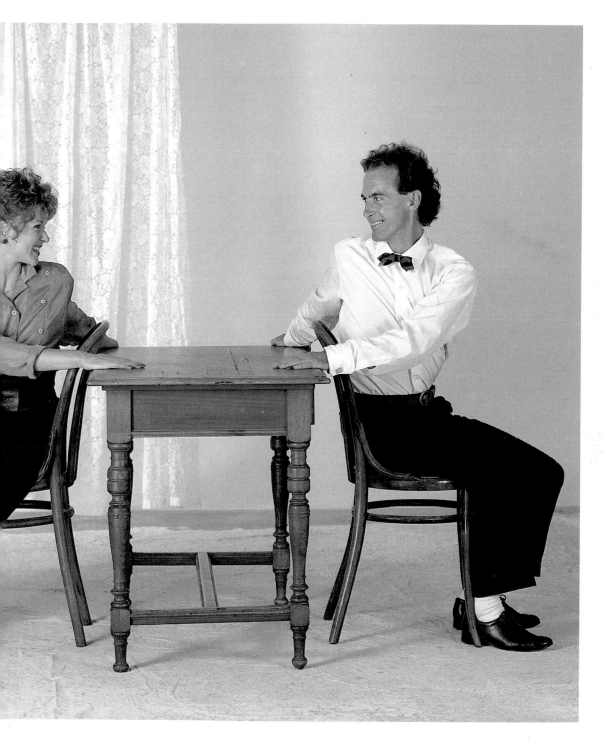

4 THAT DARNED PENCIL

Once again, the pencil slips out of your hand and rolls under the chair, and you don't particularly want to look for it down on your knees. Now is the time for a flexible spine and expandable back muscles.

When sitting on a chair, are you able to reach the floor with both hands?

How To Do the Exercise

- Sit down on the very front edge of a chair with both lower legs aligned vertically with the chair legs spread to the width of your hips. Then bend your upper body forward and reach towards the floor with your hands.
- Are your lower legs in vertical position? It is important to hold them in this manner while bending forward, so that you don't tip over.
- At the end of the exercise slowly straighten up so that you don't feel dizzy.

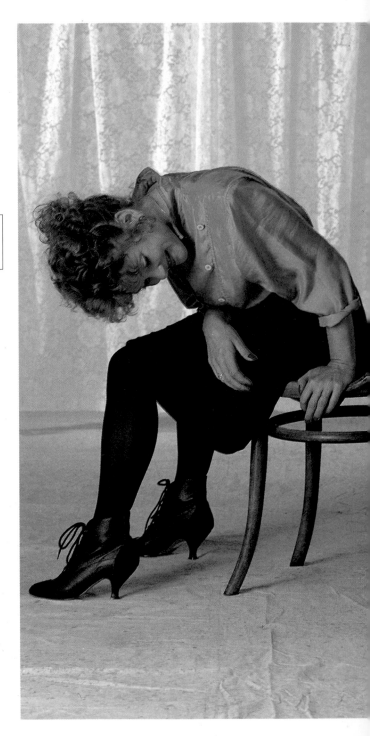

Not Yet Achieved	Passed	Good	Very Good
Exercise 8 in the 3-Stars program covers this muscle group	The fingers of both hands touch the floor without any problems	Both palms touch down on the floor next to the feet	Both palms touch down on the floor a foot behind the heels

5 A BIG STEP

Do you have a hard time swinging your leg across the saddle of your bicycle? Is your stride long enough to jump over a puddle without getting wet? In cases such as these, it is very useful to have a flexible muscular system in the upper thighs.

With this exercise, you can find out how wide your stride is.

> *Are you able to touch the floor with your fingertips while stretching your legs and doing a split?*

How To Do the Exercise

• At first, do the split while keeping your upper body erect, but go only as far as you can without effort. Be careful if the ground is slippery.
• Then slowly bend your upper body down towards the floor.
• Are both knees still stretched?
• Are you able to stay down for a couple of seconds?
• Complete the exercise by first slowly raising the upper body and then by coming out of the split.
• Even if your leg muscles are very stiff, you can still try this exercise. Try to make wider splits each time. At first, try to touch the floor with both palms and work your way up to your elbows.

Once again, don't feel satisfied with merely passing the test. You do not have to achieve a split immediately, but you should be a step towards progress.

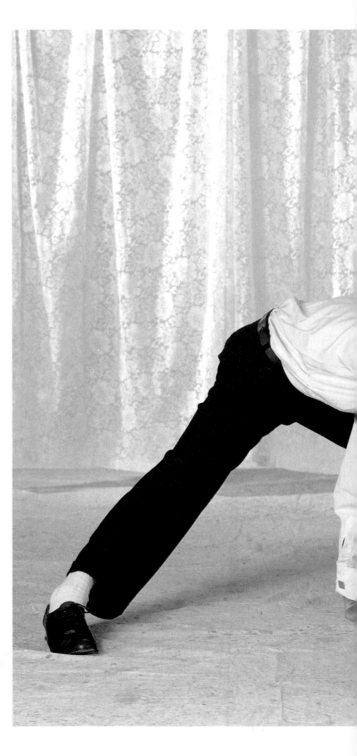

Not Yet Achieved	Passed	Good	Very Good
Exercises 4 and 5 in the 3-Stars program	Both hands touch the floor	The heels of both hands touch the floor	Both elbows rest on the floor

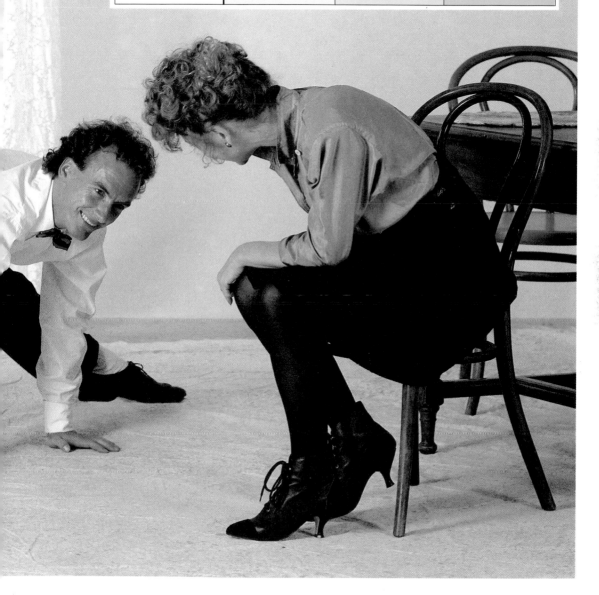

YOUR STRENGTHS AND WEAKNESSES IN AN OVERVIEW

The following table shows you all the test exercises and their effects at a glance, so that you can see where your personal weak spots are and find the right exercises for them in the 3-Stars Program.

When you have chosen your exercises, you will perform them 4 times during your workout, instead of the usual 2 times. Or you can repeat the exercises two more times at the end of your workout. Also, try to hold the stretching position a little longer, even if these exercises are the ones that you will have a difficult time in doing. This way you can make up for these weak areas and you can reach your goal of a balanced flexibility.

Test Situation Not Yet Achieved	Your Weak Spot	Remedy
The shoelace test	Flexibility of the rear leg muscles	Exercises 7 & 8
Scratching your back	Flexibility of the chest and breathing muscles	Exercise 2
Reaching for the files	Pliancy of the back and spine	Exercise 9
That darned pencil	Flexibility of the back muscles	Exercise 8
A big step	Flexibility of the inner upper-thigh muscles	Exercises 4 & 5

THE 3-STARS PROGRAM

The 3-Stars Program consists of a series of three steps that increase in difficulty and have ten exercises each:

1   The soft program for beginners
2   The extended program for demanding exercisers
3   The expanded program for experienced exercisers

Each step represents a complete, well-rounded training program. The ten exercises systematically take into consideration all important muscle groups in accordance with a balanced flexibility training and are brought into line with each other concerning sequence.

The text accompanying each exercise consists of three parts:
• a short basic description of the exercise
• an explanation of the effect
• 3 quality stars for doing the exercise better.

It also includes:
• explanations concerning the execution of the exercises
• hints concerning intensification of the exercise
• possible variations

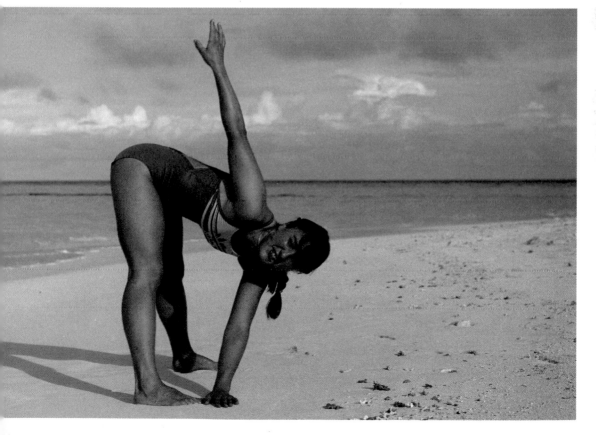

HOW TO BEGIN

When learning each new exercise, first familiarize yourself with the description and the accompanying pictures. Then read the second part, which explains the expected effects of each exercise, because each stretch can only be done correctly and experienced properly when you know which regions will be stretched and why you actually turn and bend and pull one way and not the other.

When you become familiar with the reasoning behind an exercise, you will later be able to use that information to train more independently. This way, you can explore your body completely individually.

Instructions to help you begin experimenting with an exercise are given in the quality-star sections of the programs. Here, you will find some important instructions concerning stretching positions and how each exercise can be further intensified and varied.

Should Experienced Exercisers Start with the Soft Program?

Even if you already know some of the exercises and you are not a sports newcomer, start with the beginner's program because each successive program is based on complete familiarity with the program that preceded it. And anyway, the beginner's program, when done intensively and with concentration, is not so easy even for the experienced sportsperson.

Each exercise is only as good as its performance.

How Are the 3 Steps Based on Each Other?

The **Beginner's Program** intentionally consists of very simple and elementary exercises, some of which probably even absolute sports newcomers already know, perhaps from physical education class in school.

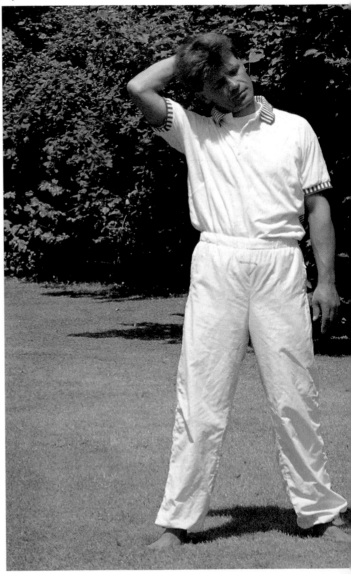

In the **Extended Program,** which is for more demanding exercisers, the simple exercises are again worked through, but, as the name indicates, they are extended. It is important, and this should be stressed over and over again, that you familiarize yourself with the beginner's program.

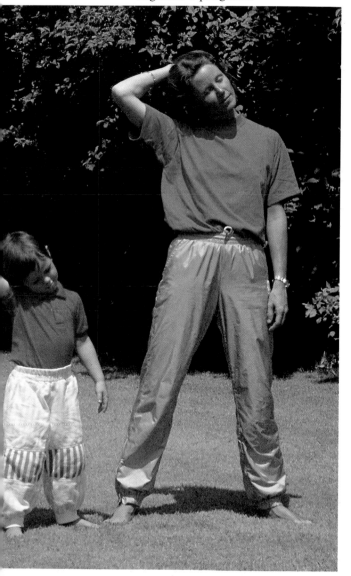

The exercises are taken even further in the **Expanded Program,** and, when you have completed this step, you will be surprised at what was hidden in the beginner's step. By following the step system, you will achieve steady progress in your training program.

How Long Should You Stick with a Program?

It is difficult to give a definite time frame for each step, because the amount of time it takes to master a step largely depends on the respective level that you started out with, on the frequency of your exercising, and of course, on your individual progress. Nevertheless, here are some minimal hints:

It's a good idea to stay with the beginner's program for at least four weeks in order to get to know the basic pattern of the presentation and the description.

When your demands grow and you become impatient to see the next pages, take the Flexibility Test one more time. Did you really improve that much or did you simply get curious? If you still have difficulties, maybe you should think about going through the basic exercises again. Do not overestimate yourself and try to keep your ambition within limits.

Also, if individual exercises of a particular program still give you problems, it makes sense to remain at that level, because the object is to reach a balanced level of flexibility throughout your body, and not, for example, to have extreme flexibility in your legs and at the same time have weak shoulder muscles. By the way, this is a common deficiency in the performance

PROGRAMS

training in many kinds of sports—only the body parts that are needed for the respective technique of the sport are especially trained.

In contrast to such performance training, your goal is a harmonic flexibility of the whole body!

Once again, it should be stressed, these are minimum time suggestions! It is more important that you develop a feeling for your body and that you allow this feeling to determine your progress than to worry about timing. When a particular training program has become second nature to you, and you feel that you want to be more challenged, then the time has come to switch to the next program.

On the other hand, if you have taken a long break or if you have been sick, you might want to proceed a little bit slower. It is really no disaster to go back a few pages and to repeat the old exercises one more time.

Should You Warm Up Before Stretching?

Yes and no.

What does this mean?

For example, if you limber up by running or walking for 5 to 10 minutes before stretching, it will provide the big advantage of warming up the muscular system, thus making it more stretchable. After that the stretching exercises can be done more intensively, without risk of injury. And of course the effects of the exercises will be greatly increased.

However, it is possible to start without warming up. The individual programs are based on each other in such a way that the first exercises are easier and at the same time serve as a warm-up.

By the Way, Do You Play Tennis, or Maybe Volleyball, Soccer, or Squash?

From your physical education class at school, you will probably remember the old principle: Warm up before doing sports! This is especially true for sports played with a partner or a team, because the concentration is usually focused on the game and the partner(s). In such cases, the heat of the event usually causes you to forget your physically determined limits.

Well, how about **stretching** to warm up? The programs are excellent for this purpose, instead of, or, at best, in combination with the limbering up run. Because stretching:

- increases the blood-circulation in the muscle tissue and thereby warms the stretched muscles
- prepares strained muscles for the stress of exercise
- provides the opportunity to free yourself from everyday problems and open yourself up to performance, fun, or play.

Stretching to Cool Off

Gentle stretching is recommended not only before doing sports but also afterwards, because it will help to prevent sore muscles and soothe those that are already sore. The program exercises are ideal for this as well, because:

- they stretch exhausted and strained muscles, thus preventing cramps caused by stress
- they supply muscle fibres with blood and accelerate the removal of waste products of the metabolism
- they not only relax the body, but also the mind

ORGANIZATION AND FOCUS OF THE EXERCISES IN THE 3 PROGRAMS

Exercise	Beginner's Program	Expanded Program and Intensification	Extended Program
1	Lateral neck muscles	Intensified stretching through hand guidance	Intensified stretching through counter-pulling with the shoulders
2	Chest and breathing muscles	Added minor stretching of the lateral trunk and shoulder muscles	Increased stretching of the lateral trunk and shoulder muscles
3	Rear neck muscles	Added stretching of the back muscles	Additional stretching of the muscular system of the posterior
4	Inner and rear upper-thigh muscles	Intensified stretching, including twisting of the upper body	Increased twisting of the upper body
5	Inner and rear upper-thigh muscles	Intensification of the stretch	Further intensification of the stretch
6	Front hip-portion and rear upper-thigh muscles	Intensified stretch	Intensification of the upper-thigh exercise
7	Rear upper-thigh and calf muscles	Intensification through alternating hand positions	Extension through incorporation of calf muscles
8	Rear upper-thigh muscles	Increased stretching through closing the legs	Further intensification by crossing the legs
9	Trunk and spine muscles	Intensified stretch of the trunk muscles	Supplementation through stretching the leg muscles
10	Calf muscles	Intensification by using exercise aids	Additional stretching of the front shinbone muscles and the back part of the foot

1 THE GENTLE PROGRAM FOR BEGINNERS EXERCISE 1

Stand with legs slightly spread and let both arms hang in a relaxed manner at your sides. Slowly tilt your head to the right towards your shoulder, while looking straight ahead, and remain in this position for about 20 seconds. Then roll your head forward and to the left, holding it towards your left side for 20 seconds.

The Exercise Effect

Before you begin stretching, really let your arms hand totally relaxed—this way your shoulders will sink down. At the same time, exhale and inhale slowly and steadily and try to calm your body with this first small introductory exercise. Of course this stretch can also be done while sitting.

3 Quality Stars

• Make sure that the head moves down towards the shoulder, not the other way around. Pull both shoulders consciously back a little and push your breastbone forward and upward. Only when standing upright can this exercise affect the right part of the body.

• During the stretch, pull your chin an inch farther in towards your neck—that way, the stretch will provide some exercise for the front neck muscles. When the chin is forward and down, the stretch moves increasingly towards the rear part of the neck.

• The stretch will be more intensive if you also pull down on the shoulder opposite the direction of the stretch.

EXERCISE 2

Hold both hands above the head while in a standing position with your legs slightly spread. Interlock your fingers, turn your palms upward, and fully extend your arms. As with all the exercises, hold the stretch for about 20 seconds.

The Exercise Effect

This stretching is for the muscular system of the arms, the shoulder-girdle, and especially for the breathing muscles in the chest between the ribs.

3 Quality Stars

• In order to really feel the stretch in the chest and breathing muscles, hold your arms way back and push your chest far forward.
• Look up towards your hands.
• With this exercise, pay special attention to your breathing, keeping it calm and relaxed.

EXERCISE 3

In a standing position, grasp the
back of your head with both hands
and entwine your fingers. Then tilt
your head forward and down by
gently pressing with your hands
until your chin touches your chest.

The Effect

The exercise can also be done in a
sitting position. Together with exercise 1, it is well suited for a quick,
relaxing stretch during work, when
typical tension problems often occur in the neck and shoulder muscles.

3 Quality Stars

• Elbows and shoulders should pull
forward and down in a relaxed
manner and support the stretch of
the back part of the neck and nape
muscles.
• Vary the direction of the pull a
bit and tilt the head once to the left
and then to the right.
• The more you round your upper
body towards the front, the more
the stretch will reach the muscles
of your back that run along the
spine. This expansion of the exercise, though, should not take place
until you get to programs 2 and 3.

EXERCISE 4

In standing position with legs spread, slowly bend your upper body forward and down until your hands touch the floor. Remain here for 20 seconds.

The Effect

The stretching is meant for the muscle groups at the back side of your legs, the so-called upper-thigh-benders.

3 Quality Stars

• Do not pull down with force—let the upper body, shoulders, and arms hang totally relaxed and let the force of gravity do the work at first. Concentrate on the stretch of the leg muscles and do the stretch very carefully.
• Set the feet apart far enough so that the hands touch the floor without problems or discomfort.
• Both legs should remain stretched for the entire time.

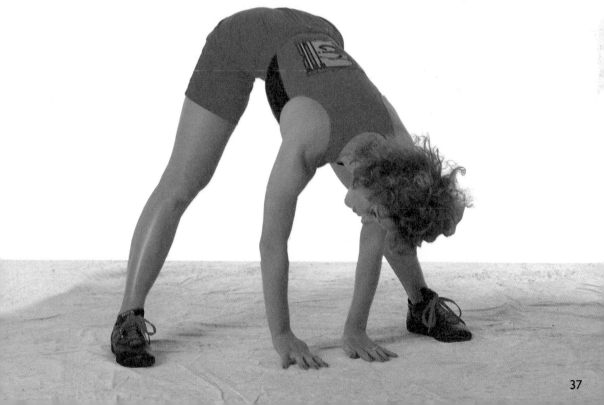

EXERCISE 5

Standing with your legs widely spread, bend your left knee until you feel a stretch in your right upper-thigh muscles. Both hands should rest on your left upper thigh. Switch sides and repeat.

The Effect

Again, go slowly into this stretch position, because the inner and rear leg muscles are often weak spots for beginners as well as for trained sportspeople.

3 Quality Stars

• The upper body should remain as erect as possible and the posterior should not move backwards. So pull your hips actively forward. The tips of the toes should point slightly outwards.
• Once you get used to the first stretch, very tentatively try the exercise again but push your feet increasingly further apart.
• The stretch emphasis can be changed by turning your upper body alternately towards the right or the left. Try it!

EXERCISE 6

In a kneeling position, move your left leg with the knee bent, in front of your body and place your hands on either side of your left foot. Slowly move your left knee forward, until you are in a comfortable stretch. Remain in this position about 20 seconds and then switch to the other side.

The Effect

The stretch will be felt on the back side of the bent leg as well in the front hip area of the stretched leg. Where you personally will feel the most stretching will depend on your individual flexibility. Different people will experience this exercise completely differently.

3 Quality Stars

• Under no circumstances should pains from pressure on the knee interfere with the stretch. Therefore, practice on a carpet or put a pillow under your knee.
• Raise your upper body and consciously push your shoulders back. Head up!
• With an erect posture, your hip will pull increasingly downward, thereby intensifying the stretch.

EXERCISE 7

In a kneeling position, move your left leg forward and place your foot on the floor so that the upper thigh of the kneeling leg is in a vertical position. Place both hands on the left leg, carefully bend the upper body forward, and remain there for 20 seconds. Repeat several times and then switch legs.

The Effect

The back side of the extended upper thigh is stretched. You will probably realize that the exercises are getting a bit more difficult in the middle of the program. If you have difficulties with this exercise, you are by no means alone. But that does not mean that you should put up with this fact.

3 Quality Stars

• Set the front leg a bit to the side so that you have no problems holding your balance.
• Keep the knee stretched! Do not bend the upper body forward too far.
• Try to release the tension of the stretch by breathing calmly and deeply. The body relaxes increasingly when exhaling.

EXERCISE 8

> In a sitting position, spread your stretched legs and then bend your upper body forward, reaching out with your hands.

The Effect

This exercise, which you probably know well, seems to be impossible to achieve for many beginners, because it requires, when done to perfection, the ability to spread the legs and also flex the back leg muscles to a high degree. But by exercising on a regular basis, sports newcomers and older people can still achieve good progress and thus gain more flexibility.

3 Quality Stars

• Do not pretend to bend the upper body forward by desperately pulling your head down. Imagine that there is a thread attached to your belly button, that pulls you forward. The stretch will only have the desired effect if you stretch the hip joint.
• First, spread your legs as far as possible and only then bend your upper body forward. Make sure that you do it with special feeling and patience.
• The knees should remain extended throughout the stretch.

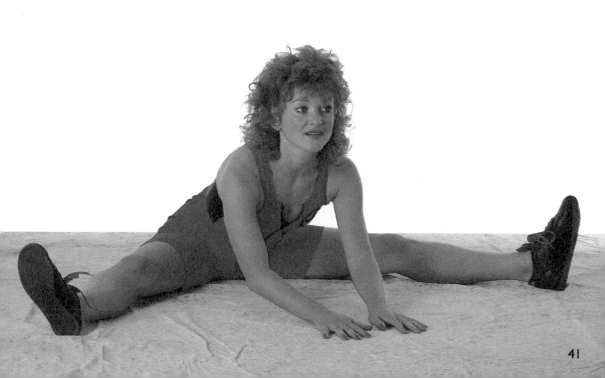

EXERCISE 9

In a sitting position, slightly bend your knees, keeping both feet flat on the floor and parallel to the hips. Keep your back straight. With your left hand, reach for your right knee, and reach behind your back with your right hand, and turn your upper body slowly to the right. Slowly untwist and do the left.

The Effect

In this "corkscrew" position, the upper body and back-spine are being stretched. Thus the exercise is good for the vertebrae and interarticular disks (meniscus) as well as for the whole muscular system of the trunk. Furthermore, the aid to your breathing can be consciously felt.

3 Quality Stars

• In order to be able to do the turn optimally, the back should be as straight as possible. Then induce the twist from the area of the lumbar (pelvis) vertebra and then continue the turning movement up into the thoracic (chest) vertebrae and then to the cervical (neck) vertebrae. When releasing the stretch you reverse the procedure. You begin by turning the head and then you release the twist, vertebra by vertebra, downwards.

• Support yourself when in the "corkscrew"—press against your knee with your hand and, with the other hand, move it inch by inch further behind your back.

• Your shoulders should be perpendicular to your pelvis. Therefore, pull the rear shoulder actively backward and the front shoulder in the direction of the knee. Do you feel the stretch in the shoulder girdle?

EXERCISE 10

Stand in a stride-position, with your right foot before your left, about one arm length away from a table or wall and support yourself with your hands. Stretch the left leg by pressing the left heel to the floor and hold it there for 20 seconds. Then switch sides.

The Effect

It is important that the toe of the rear foot of the leg points forward towards the wall, because only in that position will the back calf muscles and the Achilles tendon be affected by the stretch.

3 Quality Stars

• Vary the width of the stride position and the distance to the wall, until you have found a comfortable stretch.

• You can also do the stretch by slowly pushing your hip forward, without lifting your heel from the floor.

• Always keep the back leg totally stretched. Suppose that the beginner's program has now in fact very gently but surely become an essential part of your daily routine. The stretches are no longer a big effort, and you have no problems at all doing the individual exercises. As a matter of fact, your demands are growing gradually. Then there is no reason to continue— the next program is already waiting for you. You only have to flip to the next page.

2 THE EXTENDED PROGRAM FOR DEMANDING EXERCISERS

Have you mastered the exercises in the beginner's program? Do you have the feeling that your demands are gradually growing and that you are no longer challenged by the exercises? Then the path is open for the next, more demanding program: Each individual exercise is extended and designed more demandingly, but that way it is also more interesting. Compare the former exercise 5 with exercise 5 of the extended program: An intensified upper-thigh-stretch is added to the simple bend of the upper body.

EXERCISE 1

Stand with legs slightly spread and your head towards the left shoulder. Then touch the head with the left hand and gently and carefully support the tilt of the head—by doing so you will support the stretch. The upper body should remain erect. Hold the stretch for 20 seconds and switch sides.

The Effect

The neck muscles are particularly prone to tenseness, which leads to manifold ailments. Therefore, take your time for this seemingly "small" exercise. Before you begin: relax your shoulders, exhale deeply, and this way release all tension. Only in this way can you fully enjoy this and the following exercises. This exercise can also be done in a sitting position, for example, at the desk to relax the neck muscles.

3 Quality Stars

• Caution! Under no circumstance should you forcefully press the head down. It is certainly the point of this exercise to intensify the stretch of the lateral neck muscles, but not to the point of muscle strain.
• Try using your hand to alter the direction of the stretch and thus its emphasis.
• When the free arm also pulls down on the head, the stretch becomes more intense.

EXERCISE 2

Stand with spread legs and stretch your right arm upward while bending your upper body to the left. Rest your left hand on your left leg. Hold this position about 20 seconds and then switch sides.

The Effect

The exercise looks easier than it really is. Without your knowing it, your body will often turn to the side, or your hip will swing to the side. The intended effect on the lateral trunk and shoulder muscles gets lost that way. You may be able to control this if you do the exercise in front of a mirror.

3 Quality Stars

• Begin the exercise by reaching far up with the stretched arm, creating a primary stretch on the side of your body. Only then should you bend your upper body to the side and extend the stretch into your waist. Your stretched arm should act as an extension of your upper body and your head, which should continue this lateral stretch, not simply hang loosely.
• Both legs remain stretched, with both feet pressed firmly onto the floor and the weight equally distributed between them.
• Pull your right shoulder back as you bend your body sideways so that the arm pulls a bit more behind your head. Do you feel the stretch wandering into the side of your body and your chest area?

EXERCISE 3

In a standing position, grasp the back of your head with both hands and interlock your fingers. With slight pressure from the hands, bend your head forward and down and then round your upper body.

- After doing the exercise, slowly straighten your back completely and pull both elbows far back.
- When straightening up, inhale deeply. You can repeat this exercise several times in coordination with your breathing exercise.

The Effect

The upper body is not bent down with this exercise. Otherwise, the stretch will affect the leg muscles instead of the back muscles. That will happen in subsequent exercises.

3 Quality Stars

- Begin the exercise with a tilt of the head, feel the stretch in the upper neck area, and then slowly roll the upper body forward until the stretch spreads down to the lower part of your spine.

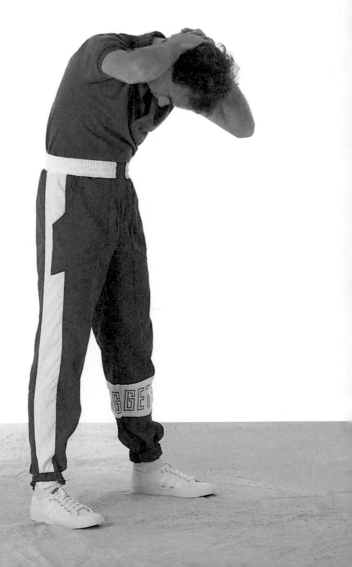

EXERCISE 4

Stand with legs spread and bend your upper body far down. Grasp your right foot with your left hand and stretch your right arm up and over your back. Hold this position for 20 seconds. Switch sides.

The Effect

Through the strong bend of the upper body, the muscles on the back sides of your legs are stretched. The further you spread your legs, the more the muscles of the inner side of the legs will be stretched as well.

3 Quality Stars

• The left shoulder should reach for the right knee, and the right shoulder should pull backwards and up with the arm. Thus, in addition to the stretching of the leg, you also stretch the whole trunk area.
• Look at your upper hand, twisting your head all the way down to the neck vertebrae.
• The legs always remain stretched.

EXERCISE 5

In a wide split position, rest both hands on the floor and slowly bend the right knee until you feel a stretch on the left inner side of the upper thigh. Hold it for 20 seconds and then switch sides.

The Effect

When you have the feeling that you are especially stiff in these parts of your body, this will serve as an incentive to work a bit more on your weak spots. After all, balanced freedom of motion is the goal.

3 Quality Stars

• The emphasis here is on going into the position slowly, in order to avoid stress.

• After a first feel of the stretch, it is safe to proceed a little further. But remember, masochism has nothing to do with stretching!

• Support the bent leg on the inner side with your elbow and gently push it backwards. When the knee is approximately above the tip of the toe, that means that it is not tilted forward and the stretch becomes noticeably more intensive.

EXERCISE 6

From a kneeling position, set the right foot forward. Rest both hands on the bent right knee. Enhance the stride position until you feel a stretch. Remain in that position for 20 seconds and then switch legs.

The Effect

The more erect the upper body is, the more the stretch there will be in the front hip and leg area. This should be the main focus of this stretching exercise.

3 Quality Stars

• To straighten the upper body means to consciously pull your shoulders back, push forward with your breastbone, and keep your head straight. This way the hip will sink down best and support the stretch.

• You should have your back instep on the floor and your front foot should be standing with the entire sole flat on the floor. You also can support yourself on the side with your hand in case you have trouble keeping your balance.

• Again and again, especially when you have difficulty, very consciously try to relax. Breathe calmly and deeply, maybe close your eyes and concentrate completely on yourself and the stretch feeling.

EXERCISE 7

In a kneeling position, stretch the right leg forward and set your foot down. The upper thigh of the kneeling leg should be almost vertical. Set your hands to the left and right of the right foot, and slowly bend forward your upper body. Remain there for 20 seconds. Then switch leg positions.

The Effect

As in exercise 7 of the beginner's program, here again the back part of the leg muscles are the main focus. But with the changed position of the hands it is intensified.

3 Quality Stars

• Before the upper body pulls forward, position your pelvis rather upright. That is, while the right leg is being stretched forward, the right hip should be pulled back a bit so that the axle of the hip and the stretched leg form a "T".
• The upper body should lean forward to the tip of the toe and not down to the leg. The leg should remain as straight as possible.
• Enhance the stride position by shifting the front foot further forward. But pay attention to the knee: The leg should remain stretched throughout the entire time.

EXERCISE 8

In a sitting position, with stretched and closed legs, pull your upper body forward. Your hands should reach forward to the tips of your toes.

The Effect

At first sight, this exercise may seem easier on the rear upper-thigh muscles than the one in the first program. But it is only really effective when the bend forward comes from the hip joint. Pay attention very carefully here to the Quality-Stars.

3 Quality Stars

• Before you pull the upper body downward in a tense manner, let a feeling of heaviness come over you that loosely pulls your shoulders and arms down. Then give in to this feeling of heaviness with a forward bend until tension in your upper thigh counteracts the stretch.
• The legs should remain as stretched as possible, even if this prevents you from bending very far forward with your upper body.
• Avoid stooping. Look straight ahead and try to lean with the tip of your nose towards your toes and with your belly button towards your upper thighs.

EXERCISE 9

In a sitting position on the floor, bend your knee into an angle, placing your foot next to your left knee. The left leg is straight. Your left hand should reach to your right knee, your right arm should reach far behind your body. Through gentle pressure with the left hand against the right knee, turn your body to the right and remain there for 20 seconds.

The Effect

After three exercises for the flexibility of the leg muscles and the hip joint, here is an exercise that includes the trunk muscles.

3 Quality Stars

• Before you start the stretch, pull your back straight. Imagine that there are two strings fastened to you at the top of your head and at your breastbone, and they are pulling you straight like a marionette. Only then, vertebra by vertebra, begin to twist your body. Both hips and the straight leg should stay in contact with the floor, because the spine should only twist along the lengthwise axis.

• Twist the shoulder so far that it is perpendicular to the pelvis. This exercise also makes the joints of the shoulder girdle flexible.

• You can intensify the exercise by crossing your left elbow over your right knee, so that you left underarm rests on your right upper thigh.

EXERCISE 10

In stride position, right foot before left foot, stand about an arm-length distance away from a wall or table, and prop yourself against it with both hands. Place a book under the tip of your left foot and stretch the left leg and pull the left knee towards the floor.

The Effect

The tip of the set back foot points forward, because this way the stretch starts on the Achilles tendon and the rear calf muscles. This exercise is particularly good if you run often, because it balances the high stress on the calf muscles.

3 Quality Stars

• The weight should be on your front leg, which is bent, so that you can balance the pressure with your heel against the floor.
• The back leg should be fully stretched so that the stretch reaches into the outer calf muscles. If you bend your knee a little bit, the under layer of the calf muscles are increasingly stretched. Both variations are good stretches that make sense.
• By pushing the hip forward, the stretch becomes more intensive.

By doing the Beginner's and Extended programs, you have now become thoroughly acquainted with the structure of the exercises with their extensions and intensifications. You also realize how small variations can make a position substantially more exhausting and also, the difference between doing an exercise thoughtlessly or executing it with concentration on all the subtleties, thus discovering the hidden effects and problems of a stretch. If, despite all this, the demanding program is no longer demanding enough, move on to the expanded program for experienced exercisers. It will take you another step in the direction of greater flexibility.

3 THE EXPANDED PROGRAM FOR EXPERIENCED EXERCISERS EXERCISE 1

In a standing position, with legs spread slightly, put your hands behind your back, interlock your fingers and extend your arms. Bend your head to the right, continuing to look straight ahead.

The Effect

By positioning your arms this way, your shoulders are pulled downwards and fixed there. This way they offer good resistance for stretching the lateral hand muscles.

3 Quality Stars

• Stretch the arms and elbows and pull the interlocked hands down until the shoulder blades are close to each other.
• With a slight change of the chin position, you can work different parts of the muscular system of the neck. Let the stretch wander.
• Push the chest forward, so that you can also stretch the breathing muscles.

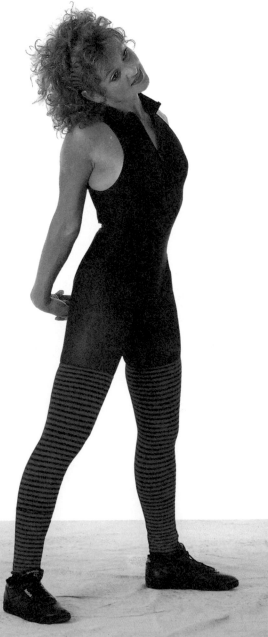

EXERCISE 2

In a standing position, with slightly spread legs, stretch your right arm upward and put your lower arm into an angle. Let your right hand hang loosely down behind your neck, and reach with your left hand for the tip of your right elbow, then pull it to the left. The upper body should follow the direction of the pull.

The Effect

The exercise has two effects: The muscles of the upper arm are stretched, and the sideways bend of the upper body stretches the side muscles.

3 Quality Stars

• Despite the stretch of the breathing muscles, do not interrupt your normal breathing.
• In the side bend, pull the elbow a bit backwards—do you feel the difference?
• Head up! The head pulls the spine diagonally to the side.

EXERCISE 3

In a standing position, with legs spread parallel to the hips, hold onto the back part of your head with both hands and interlock your fingers. With slight support of the hands, bend your head and upper body forward and bend your legs slightly.

The Effect

Despite the similarity to Exercise 3 in the first two programs, this exercise has a different focus—the back is completely rounded and the stretch of the straight back muscles is continued down into the muscles of the posterior.

3 Quality Stars

• Direct a lot of feeling towards the pressure in your hands. The neck-vertebrae area is a very sensitive zone, and under no circumstances should it be strained too much.
• The elbow tips should pull forward and down in a relaxed manner.
• After completing the exercise, straighten your back and pull both elbows backwards. At the same time, inhale deeply.

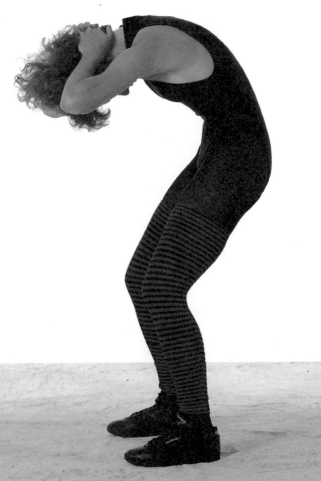

EXERCISE 4

From a wide split position, bend the upper body down. Reach with your right hand to your left foot, bend your left knee and pull your left arm far backwards over your side. Switch sides.

The Effect

By bending your leg, the twist action of the upper body is enhanced, in contrast to the same exercise in the second program, and the entire muscular system of the trunk and the shoulder girdle is stretched comprehensively. In addition, the muscular system of the legs is included in the stretch.

3 Quality Stars

• The stretch position is relatively complex: Try and vary it a bit, until you have found a position that is comfortable for you.
• Pull the right shoulder actively towards the bent left knee and pull the left shoulder far back. Look at your upper hand; this way you will achieve an optimal turn of the upper body.
• The further you set your feet apart, the stronger the stretch becomes for the leg muscles.

EXERCISE 5

In a wide split position, bend your right leg and push your posterior down as far as possible. The point of the left foot should be turned up, and both hands should rest on the floor.

The Effect

This stretching exercise is certainly quite advanced and represents an excellent stretch for the inner and back leg muscles.

3 Quality Stars

- The bent right knee should not tilt forward. Therefore, support it with your elbow and push it backwards. Put your weight onto the entire sole of your right foot.
- Turn the point of the left foot upward. This way the leg is turned outwards at the hip joint and the stretch is shifted from the inner side of the leg more to the back part of the upper thigh area.
- Again, have patience when doing this exercise—"iron will" does not lead to the goal here.

EXERCISE 6

From a kneeling position, place your left foot in front of you and enlarge the stride position until a stretch is experienced. The left hand should rest to the left of the body on the floor, and the right arm should be stretched and pulled far upwards and diagonally backwards. Then switch sides.

The Effect

By bringing the stretched arm backwards, the stretch is extended along the front of the upper side of the stretched leg to the upper thigh area; that means the stretch is spread to the entire right side of the body.

3 Quality Stars

• The stretching position is relatively complex: Try and vary it a bit until you have found a complete stretch.
• Actively pull the right shoulder towards the bent left knee and pull the left shoulder far backwards. Look at your upper hand; this way you will achieve an optimal turn of the upper body.
• The further you set your feet apart, the stronger the stretch of the muscles will be.

EXERCISE 7

From a kneeling position, stretch your right leg forward and place the heel on the floor. The upper body should bend forward, and be supported by the right hand. The left hand should grasp the point of the right foot and pull it towards the shin. Hold, repeat several times, and switch legs.

The Effect

Through the forward bend of the upper body, the back part of the upper thigh muscles are stretched. By turning up the point of the foot, the stretch is increased, as is the muscular system of the calves.

3 Quality Stars

• Seek a stable balance when positioning your body, because you will tense up the muscles that you are trying to stretch, making it more difficult to do the exercise.

• Only very gently pull the point of the foot towards you. The knee should really remain stretched, otherwise the effect of the stretch will be lost.

• The upper body should reach more forward than down.

EXERCISE 8

In a sitting position, cross your left leg over your stretched right leg, so that the left knee rests on the right knee. Bend the upper body forward and reach with your hands to the point of the foot on the stretched leg. Switch legs and cross the right leg over the left.

The Effect

You will probably feel an increased pull at the hollow of the knee. By crossing the legs, the lower leg cannot move upwards, and this way the bending muscles on the back side of the legs are stretched intensively.

3 Quality Stars

• Before you bend your upper body forward with all your willpower, first give yourself some time to get used to the positioning of the legs, since the stretching position alone can already be quite demanding. Only then carefully move with the upper body forward.

• Again it is imperative: Bend the upper body from the hip joint—a crooked back does not have any effect on the leg muscles. Imagine that you want to touch your legs with your belly button.

• Do not let your head hang down. But just the same, do not tilt the head too much into the neck. The head should pull the spine straight and forward.

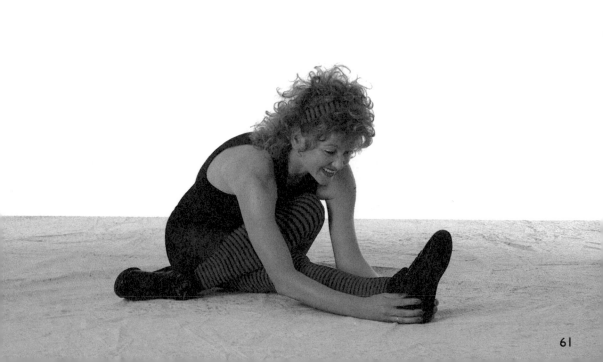

EXERCISE 9

In a sitting position, put both legs
into an angle and tilt your left leg
outward and down to the floor.
Then place your right leg on the
outside next to your left knee.
Cross the left elbow over your
right knee, and slowly turn your
upper body to the right. The right
hand should reach far behind you.

The Effect

This exercise is borrowed from
yoga, but besides the effects that
are wanted in yoga, it also provides
a good stretching of the upper body
and the leg muscles.

3 Quality Stars

• Before you start to turn your upper body, you should feel comfortable in the starting position. Both
hips should lie flat on the floor in as
relaxed a manner as possible, and
the weight should be evenly distributed on them. The back should be
pulled totally straight.
• As in Exercise 9 in the first 2 programs, the twist of the upper body
is fixed through pressure of the elbow against the knee.
• Begin the turn from the lumbar
vertebrae region, and proceed vertebra by vertebra upward to the neck
vertebrae. Try to pull the upper
body straight with the turn and to
move with the twist.

EXERCISE 10

Bend your body over and support it with both arms stretched. Your legs should also be stretched out behind you. Now bend the left knee and push the right heel towards the floor. Your left instep should rest on the floor. Hold the stretch for 20 seconds and then switch legs. Repeat several times.

The Effect

As in Exercise 10 in the first and second programs, here again the back part of the muscular system of the lower leg is stretched. By "folding over" the front foot, the front part of the foot and shinbone is stretched as well—a good balance to the calf stretch.

3 Quality Stars

• When doing the first stretch, slowly pull the heel down, because these muscles are shortened in many people, and the Achilles tendon should always be treated gently.

• Make sure that the point of the foot on your stretched leg really points forward, because only then will the exercise have the intended effect.

• Press the instep of the bent leg actively down, but without getting tense.

If you have now also mastered the program for experienced exercisers, that does not mean that you have reached your goal and that you can rest on your laurels. Flexibility and freedom to move come only with constant exercise.

To this effect, the Three-Stars Program can and will be your personal training program in the long run, and can adapt to your training level. If you can keep up with the program for experienced exercisers, then you have achieved a lot. But it is also the purpose of the 3-Stars Program to demonstrate to you the variability of stretches that seem so simple at the beginning. The exercises in this book can only present a small part of the diversity of possible body positions. If you believe that you have now really "mastered" these programs, the path is open to even further enhancement of your movements.

BREATHING AND RELAXING

BREATHING, INNER TENSION, AND MUSCLE TONE

Not only after you have walked up 5 flights is it possible for you to be out of breath. Quick, flat breathing is an unmistakable sign of inner unrest, haste, and mental imbalance. Disturbed breathing rhythm is one of the body's first reactions to a disturbance in mental equilibrium. If nothing is done about it, this tension will spread from the breathing to the entire body, and tensions in the muscular system will be the result. Surely everybody has at one time observed that, for example, under increased work pressure, the breath becomes increasingly flat, the shoulders increasingly pull upward, and finally all of the shoulder muscles cramp up.

And vice versa, tensions that begin in the muscular system soon have their effect on the breathing. Thus, tense and shortened muscles reduce the width of the movements in the thorax and limit the active area of the lungs, and consequently, the exchange of oxygen. From the breathing, the effect finally spreads into the psyche—the vicious circle closes. Deep, conscious inhaling and exhaling, on the other hand, result in a rhythmic exchange of tension and relaxation, whereby relaxation is increased with each breath. The result is a reduction of muscle tone.

In many cases, we are simply no longer capable of overcoming the outside causes of this disturbance of equilibrium, and of recovering our bodily, spiritual, and mental bal-

ance. But, as shown in the circle of effects, there is the possibility of starting with the outside signs and changing the effect. For example, we can influence our bodily tension consciously through our breathing rhythm. Thus, since breathing is a pivotal point for relaxation, bodily well-being, and performance capability, an extra breathing exercise is woven into the following chapter.

In general, stretching exercises present a good opportunity to stir the concentration onto the breathing rhythm and to practice it, when the exercises are done in a calm manner. Furthermore, you can improve the flexibility of those muscles that contribute to a deep, complete breathing.

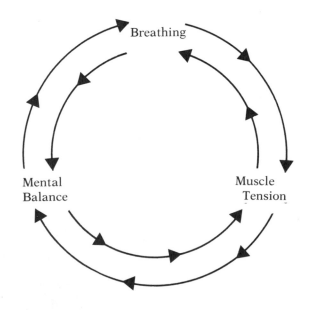

Interrelated effect of breathing, inner tension and muscle tone

Breathing

Mental Balance

Muscle Tension

WHAT DOES "COMPLETE" BREATHING MEAN?

When we speak of complete and deep breathing, we mean breathing in which all parts of the pulmonary system—from the diaphragm to the tips of the lungs—are incorporated.

The emphasis is on the so-called *belly breathing*. With this form of breathing the diaphragm, which is the lowest portion of the pulmonary system, is actively raised and lowered. When raised, the lungs' volume is reduced during exhalation; when lowering it, the area of the lungs is expanded during inhalation. On the outside, this movement of the lungs is visible as a retraction and arching of the abdominal wall. This lifting and lowering intensifies the blood circulation and massages the intestines. Through the stimulation of important nervous system points in the stomach area (solar plexus), which contributes to the complex regulation of the mood. Belly breathing contributes to a positive mood. With the so-called *breast breathing*, the central parts of the lungs are ventilated. Often this is the only active part of the breathing, especially when belly breathing is constricted by a "fashionable" tight pair of pants, or something similar.

If there is also inability to stretch the rib muscles, the oxygen exchange is considerably restricted. The breathing is "complete," when the upper parts of the lungs take part in the breathing process. One speaks of the "full-lung" breathing. This is visible when the shoulders lift and lower themselves in the breathing rhythm. It is therefore easily understandable that tense shoulder muscles impair free movement and ventilation in these areas.

In the following breathing exercise, three main parts of the lungs are ventilated intensively with oxygen.

This Is How You Can Learn "Complete" Breathing

Find a room with as much ventilation as possible, either next to an open window or outside is best. Then let your breathing rhythm progress in the following manner with this threefold exercise:

Part 1: Practice active breathing with the diaphragm in order to ventilate the lowest parts of the lungs.

Part 2: Then concentrate on the ventilation of the central parts of the lungs; that means emphasize the chest-breathing.

Part 3: Now try to let your breaths flow all the way to the tops of your lungs.

The threefold breathing exercise is an excellent introduction to your stretching program.

• because deep breathing is accompanied by a deep relaxation and your daily problems are literally blown away.

• because through psychic relaxation, physical tension in the muscles decreases and you then will be able to stretch more intensively and with more enjoyment.

You can also do this exercise separate from the stretching program. You don't need a lot of room, preparations, or start-up exercises. So, if you are in need of fresh air and fresh energy and you want to relax, then breathe deeply.

1 DIAPHRAGM BREATHING

It is best to do this and the following exercises in a standing position, because then you have the biggest freedom of movement in your chest. Place both hands on your abdomen, or, to be more specific, on your stomach area. One hand should be placed a bit above the navel, the other one a bit higher, over the diaphragm.

Each time you inhale, try to push your abdominal wall forward, so that you can feel it. That is a sign that the diaphragm has moved downward and that the lower lung area is being filled with oxygen.

When you exhale, the abdominal wall is stretched a bit, and thus the intestines are pushed inwards and the diaphragm upwards. The used air is thus actively breathed upwards and out.

Repeat this exercise 15 to 20 times, until you have really developed a feeling for the movements in this breathing method, and until you can totally become absorbed in the breathing rhythm.

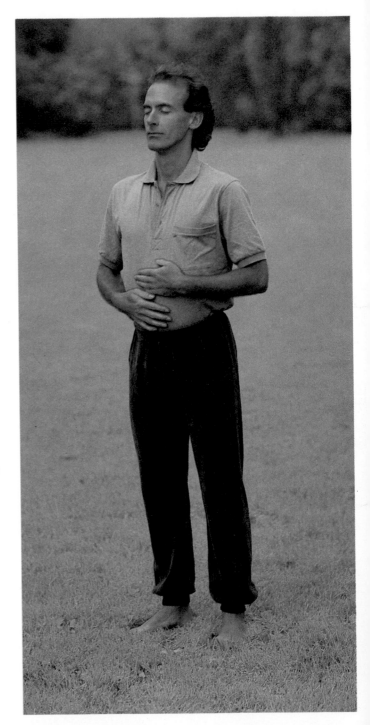

2 CHEST BREATHING

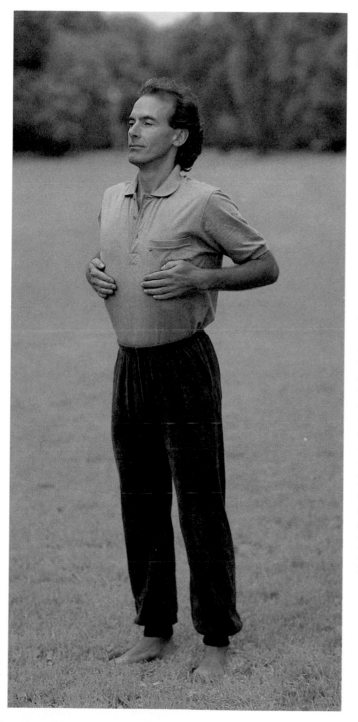

Place both hands sideways on the chest, about the height of your costal arch (the area where your lower ribs join your sternum). Now again breathe deeply and try above all to fill the middle part of your lungs with air, so that you can feel how the chest expands.

When you exhale, relax again and let the air blow out without resistance. Because this type of breathing causes the most difficulty for most people, try to concentrate on an even breathing rhythm:

• You should exhale at least as long as you inhale—try to count in your head.
• The exhaled air should flow out slowly and evenly.
• Exhale completely, but not so completely that you have to gasp for air.
• With each exhalation and inhalation, you will undergo a change between tensing up and relaxing. Enjoy to the fullest the relaxation and loosening-up when exhaling, and with each breath deepen these sensations. Repeat this exercise 15 to 20 times, before you go to the last method, the full-lung breathing.

3   FULL-LUNG BREATHING

Place both hands on your shoulders. Then try to inhale air up to the tops of your lungs. Your shoulders will automatically lift themselves a little bit upwards and backwards, which you can easily feel with your hands. When you exhale, both shoulders will sink far down and with each breath, even a bit further down. Do you feel, how quickly relaxation sets in? Inhale and exhale deeply, without holding air in-between your breaths, and let relaxation come—do not resist it. Repeat this exercise 15 to 20 times, until it "runs all by itself."

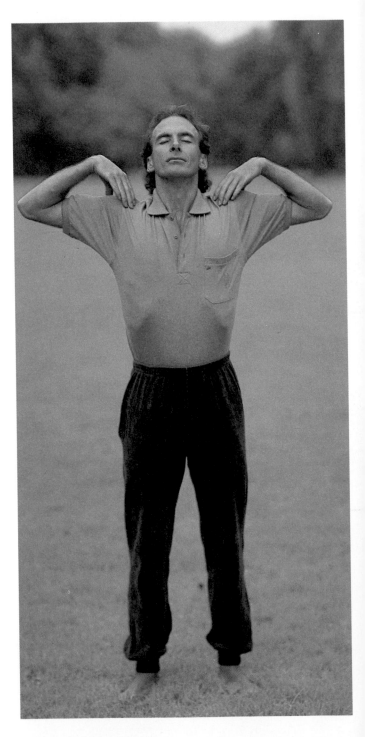

DEEP MUSCLE RELAXATION

Emotional stress, intensive "brain" work, or constant stimuli lead to increased electrochemical activity in the brain. As a result, the nerves that lead to the muscles are activated, causing them to contract and possibly cramp in the long run. These cramps often make themselves felt in the form of blood-supply problems (e.g., cold feet), difficulties in falling asleep or pains (e.g., headaches, backaches).

The following relaxation exercise, which alternates between an active tension and loosening-up of individual body parts, results in a distinct decrease of the nervous tension in the individual muscle fibres—it therefore literally helps to calm down your nerves. This form of relaxation can be learned without psychological help, and therefore presents itself as a companion to the stretching and breathing exercises, whether you want to add it to your stretches or take a break to relax in connection with your breathing exercises.

This is How You Can Relax Deeply

Take 10 minutes of your time. Lie down on a carpet in a comfortable, quiet, and well-ventilated spot. It is best to relax while lying on your back, because in that position no part of the body has to be held against the force of gravity. The arms should rest at the sides next to the body and the points of the feet should loosely tilt outwards. Pull the chin a bit in the direction of the breastbone.

Now use the following system to relax the body parts listed below:
• Tense the area for about 5 seconds until the particular muscles feel totally hard.
• Release the tension in the same muscles (again about 5 seconds).
• Now relax for 20 to 30 seconds, before you start on the next body part.

Relax the following muscle groups in this order:

Feet, legs, posterior
Stretch toes, tense lower legs and upper thighs, and squeeze posterior muscles (if you tend to get cramps on the sole of the foot, you can also pull the tips of the toes upwards).

Abdomen
Press lumbar vertebrae to the floor, let stomach muscles become hard.

Arms, shoulders.
Make a fist, stretch arms, tense chest muscles.

Neck, head, face
Pull shoulders up, press head to floor, grimace.

Remain lying on the floor a little while after tensing the last body part in order to sense how you feel.

Now you can start with your stretching program.

THE EXTRA PROGRAMS
THE CONCEPT

Exhausted? Run Down?

Do you often feel totally exhausted in the office?

On long journeys in the car, do you sometimes feel as though you were literally "run down?"

Do you regularly have difficulties trying to get going in the morning?

When you jog, do you feel "out of power" but by no means comfortably relaxed?

In such cases it is time for one of the extra programs:

1   **The extra program to wake up**
—5 exercises to get up to do in the morning in bed

2   **The extra program to "work" out**
—5 exercises to freshen up at the office

3   **The extra program for "running"**
—5 exercises to balance jogging

4   **The extra program to refuel**
—5 exercises to cheer up when driving.

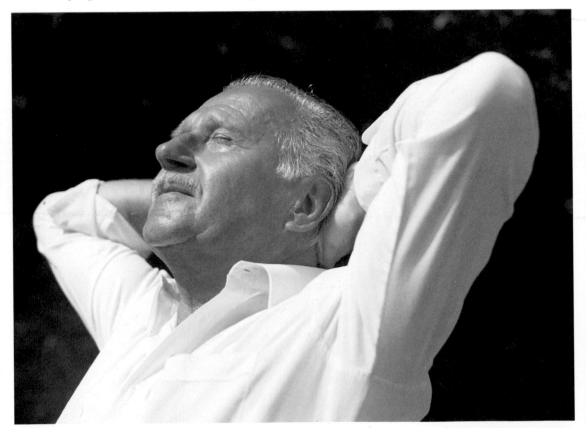

Each of the 4 extra programs is, through its choice and combination of exercises, coordinated to suit the respective situation and your needs. But that does not mean that one can or may do the exercise only then! On the contrary, you are of course free to try it out now and at any other time. Again, no preparations are necessary. You only need a couple of minutes before you quickly realize how good the little stretch in between will be for you.

Can You Combine the Exercises of the Extra Programs with the 3-Stars Program?

The extra programs are always a good idea, when you want to turn off your mind during every day routine or you want to loosen up, when the time does not seem right for an extended stretching program, or the environment does not seem suited.

But of course these "little extras" are also a supplement to the main program. For example, if you are in the mood to stretch even more intensively, you can add the 20 additional, interesting exercises of the extra programs. But be sure to extend your 3-Stars Program only when the basic exercises have become second nature to you. Too many different things are just distractions, and will prevent a relaxed, self-forgetting sinking into oneself and into the exercise. Under no circumstance should the extra programs become a substitute for your 3-Stars Program, because then the balance of the training gets lost.

What Do the Extra Programs Offer?

At the beginning of each extra program, you will find some helpful information concerning the exercise group and you will find out the main focuses of each respective exercise choice.

The 5 exercises are arranged in order, and it is therefore the most practical to stick to this order.

The description is, as in the 3-Stars Program, divided into 3 parts:
• a brief description,
• tips concerning the effects,
• three quality stars with details about the stretch position and ways to intensify and vary it.

Reserve at least 8 to 10 minutes of your time for each extra program; this way you can perform each exercise without being in a rush and easily repeat it twice. Are you not quite in such a rush? Then precede the little unit with the breathing exercises of pp. 66 to 68 to get tuned in. That helps to leave behind the rest of the world.

I THE EXTRA PROGRAM TO WAKE UP

5 Getting Up Exercises for the Morning

This little wake-up program will help make getting up easier (a little bit, anyway) and help you begin the morning with joy and enthusiasm—without radical methods such as cold water, loud music, or the usual cup of strong coffee. You may even stay in bed a little bit longer, because all exercises in this program are performed while lying down. You only have to fold the blanket a bit to the side.

But not everybody is a morning sulker. If you prefer to enjoy the day right from the beginning—wide awake and fresh—well, you can do the same exercises in this enviable frame of mind.

What Will the Exercises Do?

• They will stretch the whole body and the spine and in that way wake you up refreshingly and invigoratingly.
• They will extend and stretch the chest and breathing muscles, which will help you breathe deeper and more freely, thereby stimulating the blood supply to the brain. Good for a clear head in the morning!
• They will stretch the trunk and posterior muscles and thus stimulate the center of the body.
• They will stretch the leg muscles and make it a bit easier to get up.
• Last but not least, they will very carefully stimulate blood circulation. *Careful* is the key word. Stay

in bed and do the exercises very comfortably and relaxedly while lying down. And here's a small hint: Do not expect to be able to stretch as far early in the morning as when you do your 3-Stars program later in the day or in the evening. In the morning, the muscle tissue is less elastic, and only through movement during the course of the day does it become "softer."

Much fun with the following exercises!

EXERCISE 1

Lying on your back, bend both knees up into an angle and place your feet about ½ meter (20 inches) next to each other. Place both hands above your head, interlock your fingers, turn your palms up, and stretch your arms. Then pull both knees to the left towards the floor and at the same time stretch both hands far upwards. Move your legs to the other side and repeat the exercise.

The Effect

Just like sprawling, you stretch with both arms along the whole length of the upper body. By placing the knees to the side, you pull the stretch into the hip area and into the legs.

3 Quality Stars

• Set the feet apart far enough. The right leg, which pulls inward, should be in line with the body, thereby stretching the thigh muscles better.
• Also pull the left knee far to the side in order to stretch the inner leg muscles.
• At the same time, stretch the arms a bit higher and longer. This way you expand the lungs and chest. After the exercise relax and breathe deeply.

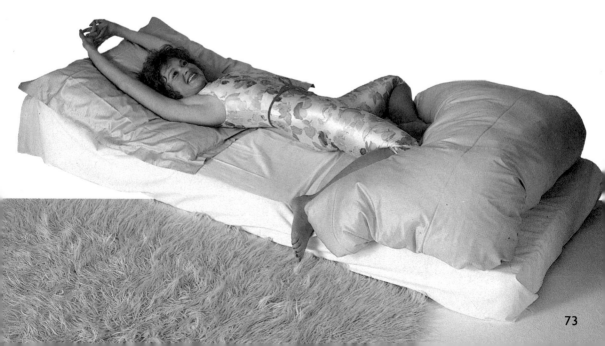

EXERCISE 2

Lying on your back, stretch your right leg vertically up into the air. Your right hand should hold your thigh at the back. Your left hand should grasp your calf. Hold your leg and try to stretch it completely. Switch legs.

The Effect

The muscles at the back side of the leg are stretched.

(Would you have realized it?)

Be careful—in the morning, the leg muscles are especially stiff.

3 Quality Stars

• Keep the arms long and relaxed. Your head and shoulders should remain calmly flat.

• The left leg should remain really stretched on the surface.

• When you feel comfortable in the position, rotate the ankle joint loosely in both directions.

EXERCISE 3

Lying on your back, bend your left leg and then fold your left knee over your right, stretched leg to the side. Your right hand should hold onto the knee and press it down; the left arm should be stretched far to the side.

The Effect

The exercise stretches the spine and is especially refreshing in the morning.

3 Quality Stars

• Do not turn your shoulder girdle with your leg, but try on the contrary to fix the left shoulder on the floor, and this way consciously counteract to the twist. In addition, look to the left.

• The long leg should remain stretched flat.

• The more you press the leg that is crossed over to the floor, the more the lateral posterior and upper-thigh muscles are stretched.

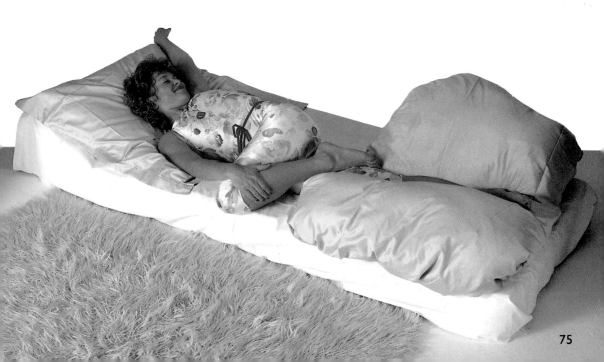

EXERCISE 4

Lying on your right side, support yourself on your right elbow; your right leg is bent back in an angle. Your left leg should be bent in an angle and your left hand should hold the left ankle and pull the heel towards the posterior.

The Effect

After the stretch for the back side of the legs in Exercise 2 and for the outer posterior muscles in Exercise 3, here is a stretch for the front part of the upper-thigh muscles.

3 Quality Stars

- Before you stretch, arrange yourself in a stable position, one in which you tilt neither backwards nor forwards. To do this, it is best to bend the lower leg backwards at an angle. You can support your upper body with your elbow or you can support your head with your hand—it is up to you how you do it.
- It is very important to push the upper hip forward, until upper thigh and body almost form a line.
- Lift your upper knee a little bit and pull the heel straight to your bottom. Lower leg and upper thigh should be parallel; this way there won't be too much strain on the knee joint.

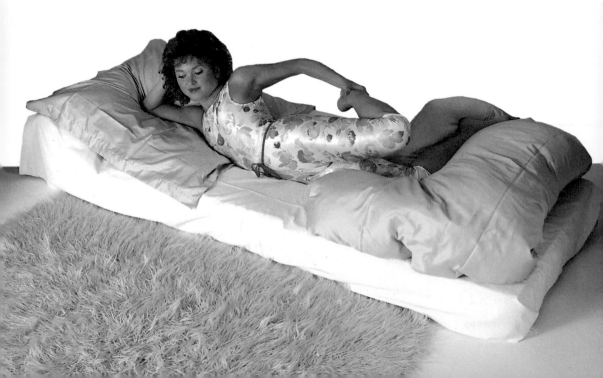

EXERCISE 5

> Lying on your belly, place both hands to the left and right of your shoulders. Slowly extend your arms and lift your upper body.

The Effect

The goal of this exercise is to stretch the front muscular system of the trunk, not to overstretch or overstress the lower part of the back. Therefore, pull the upper body more forward than upward and backward. Acrobatics are not part of stretching!

3 Quality Stars

• It is not necessary to stretch the arms completely. The main thing is that you feel the stretch along the front side of your upper body.
• Extend your arms slowly and with a lot of feeling. Pull your head to extend your spine and bend it *slightly* backwards
• Depending upon where you place the hands (more to the side or in front of the shoulders), the more or less you can pull up your upper body.

To Bring It to an End

Make a cat's back—and then out of bed!

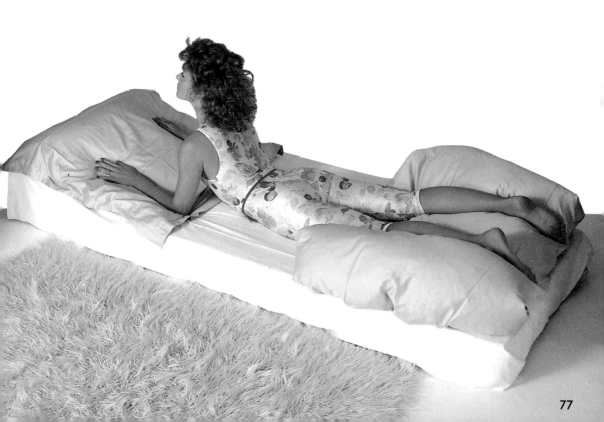

2   THE EXTRA PROGRAM TO "WORK" OUT

5   Exercises to Freshen Up at the Office

Just forget your work for a couple of minutes and stretch yourself! Rather than dispel your work energy, stretching will, on the contrary, add to it. We talk about the moment when we just cannot go on anymore, and only struggle to continue, mentally as well as physically. This is the moment when you cannot sit anymore, when your shoulders and neck get tense, and your concentration diminishes. Briefly turning off one's mind usually brings about miracles in such cases. And turning off one's mind is, without question, best done with movement and not with a cup of coffee or a piece of cake in a smoke-filled cafeteria. It is not necessary to change clothes for the following exercises because you will not sweat. Please do not be shy if you do not have your own office or if you once in a while receive a visit from colleagues or your boss. The exercises are appropriate to such circumstances. And anyway, why do you want to hide? Instead, encourage others and bring some action into the office!

The Choice of Exercises

The following five exercises concentrate on the muscle groups that often become tense or slacken when sitting for a long time:

Exercise 1—the hip-bending area
Exercise 2—the chest and trunk muscles
Exercise 3—the neck and shoulder muscles
Exercise 4—the chest and shoulder girdle muscles
Exercise 5—the back muscles of the legs

EXERCISE 1

Sit sideways on a chair, and stretch your right leg far back. Both arms should be stretched upward, the fingers interlocked and the palms turned up. The head should look up to the hands. Hold the position for about 20 seconds and then switch legs.

The Effect

This exercise stretches first the muscular system of the hip-bending area and then the muscles on the front side of the chest.

3 Quality Stars

- Sit down on the front left or right edge of the chair so that you have enough room to move your leg.
- If you pull the arms further back and if you look up to the backs of your hands, the stretch becomes even more intensive.
- Vary this exercise by stretching the point of the rear leg and by resting the instep on the floor. You will probably have to take off your shoes to do this (which your feet will most certainly welcome).

EXERCISE 2

> Sit down on a chair so that your back faces the edge of a table or desk. Both feet should be flat on the floor. Turn your upper body to the right until both hands touch the edge of the table. Pull your back straight and hold the position for 20 seconds. Then switch sides.

The Effect

You will probably already know this exercise from the flexibility test. It stretches the muscular system of the trunk and chest as well as the spine.

3 Quality Stars

• If the back of your chair is a little bit too high, then place the chair so that its back is at the side.
• The further you reach back with both hands, the stronger the stretch becomes. But make sure to keep both soles on the floor. Also, the weight should remain evenly distributed on both upper thighs. Otherwise you are cheating!
• Are you able to look at your back arm? With this turn, you can also include the muscular system of the neck in the stretch.

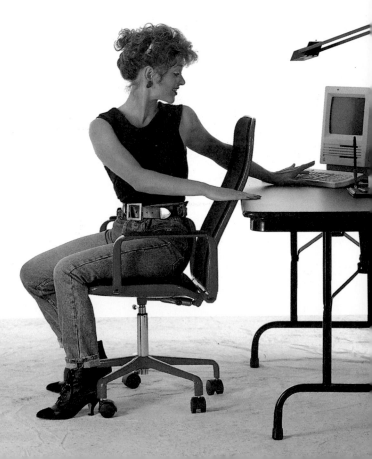

EXERCISE 3

Sitting on a chair, bend your upper body forward and down. Interlock your fingers behind your back, stretch your elbows, and pull the stretched arms forward as much as possible. At the end of the exercise, first release the hands and then roll the upper body, vertebra by vertebra, upwards again into a sitting position.

The Effect

With this exercise, you first stretch the muscular system of the shoulders and the back. In the forward bend, you stretch the posterior and the rear upper-thigh muscles.

3 Quality Stars

- Slide on the seat until you have found a position that does not present any balance problems. Spread your knees a little bit so that they do not impede the bend.
- If you lift your head a bit, then you pull increasingly down with your upper body and your stomach. The stretch of the leg muscles thereby becomes more intensive.
- Reach alternately forward and down with the arms and with the stomach.

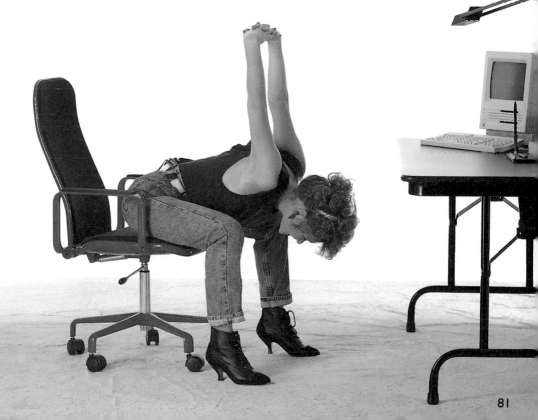

EXERCISE 4

In a standing position behind a chair, reach with both hands for the back of the chair, bend the upper body forward, and lean down until the stretched arms and the upper body are in a horizontal position. Then gently pull down with the shoulder girdle and remain there. Slowly, with a round back, roll back into an upright, standing position and repeat.

The Effect

In this exercise, the muscles that range from the ribs to the upper arms are being stretched.

3 Quality Stars

• Both arms must remain stretched, because only this way can the stretch really reach up to the arms. At the same time, do not pull your head up, but let it hang as relaxed as possible between your arms, otherwise unnecessary tension will occur in the neck.
• If the legs remain stretched, the muscles on the back side of the legs will also be flexed.
• Put the emphasis of the stretch first onto the right and then onto the left shoulder by slightly turning the upper body.

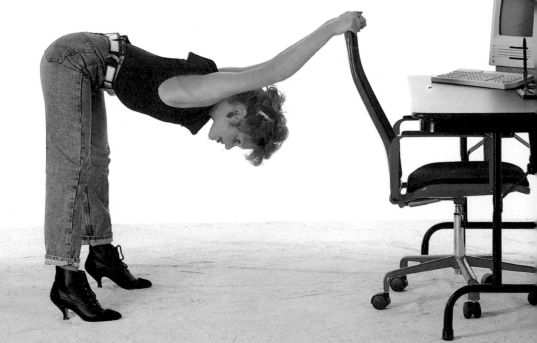

EXERCISE 5

Place the heel of the stretched left leg onto the seat of a chair. In this position, first pull the left hip a little bit backward and then bend forward with the upper body and hold the stretch there. The hands should be propped on the chair or on your knee. Slowly release and switch the legs.

The Effect

The exercise gives a strong stretch to the rear muscular system of the upper thighs and may cause difficulties for some people, because the upper-thigh muscles are often slackened from sitting a lot.

3 Quality Stars

- Bend the upper body only as far forward as you can while still keeping the leg stretched on the chair.
- The bend forward with the upper body is done from the hip joint, because only this way will the emphasis of the stretch actually reach the leg area. Therefore, do not bend forward with the head.
- The hip axle should be in a right angle to the leg that you are standing on, and should not move forward. Also, the point of the foot on the standing leg should point forward and the hip of the leg that rests on the chair should be pulled back.

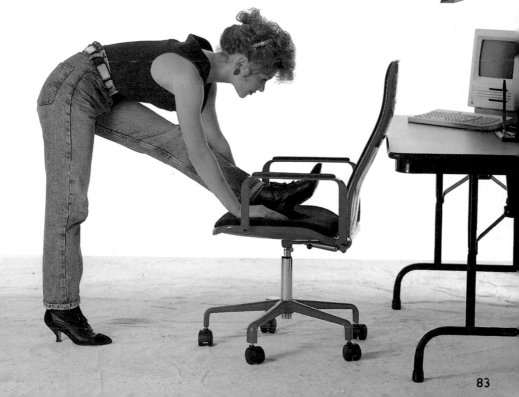

3 THE EXTRA PROGRAM FOR RUNNING

5 Exercises to Balance Jogging

Suppose you like to run. Suppose you want to get rid of stress *before* you run. Suppose you have the time and want to stretch yourself *after* jogging. Suppose you do not really know which exercises go with your running-training.

Well, here are 5 exercises that excellently supplement a running program.

If done before running, they serve to warm up as well as to prepare body and soul for the upcoming stress.

After running, you flex and loosen the muscles that have been strained while running and are therefore tense. In fact, stretches after running are particularly important, since they release tensions that may have occurred through the long strain of running.

Furthermore, the processes of regeneration in the metabolism of the muscles is supported and accelerated, which is an important factor for intensive and frequent training.

Focal Points in the Choice of Exercises

• Stretching of the arms and the shoulder girdle because these should remain loose when running, in order not to impair your breathing.

• Stretching of the spine, whereby the cartilage in the joints is relieved, which is especially important after the strain caused by kicks when running for a long time.

• Stretching of the muscular system of the upper and lower legs to balance and loosen this muscle group, which is the main stress area.

As nice as a training in fresh air is, the ground can often be uncomfortably cold and humid, making exercises in a sitting position equally uncomfortable. Therefore, use a tree as a "stretch machine"—after all, you are in the open air.

EXERCISE I

In a standing position at about 1 meter distance, the right leg is placed as high up as possible on the trunk of a tree. Now carefully shift your weight onto the bent leg, keeping your upper body straight. Prop both hands loosely onto the right knee. The right hip should push forward and down. Stay in this position for 20 seconds. Then switch legs.

The Effect

The exercise stretches the front muscular system of the hips, and upper thighs of the respective stretched leg, and the rear upper-thigh muscles and posterior muscles of the bent leg. These are the muscles that do the main work when running and therefore deserve special attention.

3 Quality Stars

• Are you standing safely? Maybe you have to correct your position somewhat, until you have a stable standing position. The points of the feet should continue to point forward and your heel should remain on the floor—that way the Achilles tendon is stretched as well.
• Keep the upper body straight and pull the hip forward.
• Of course the exercise becomes more intensive as your front leg is placed higher onto the tree.

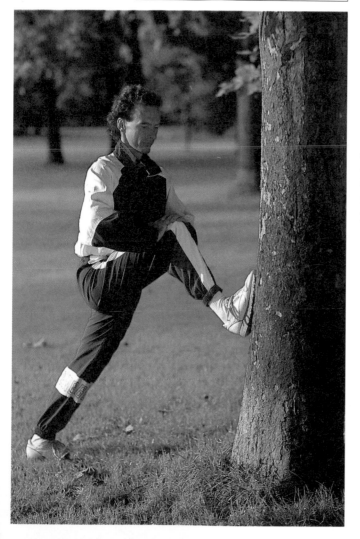

EXERCISE 2

With legs slightly spread, bend your upper body forward into a horizontal position and support yourself with stretched arms on the tree. Pull the shoulder girdle gently down and remain there. Release the stretch with a round back and repeat one more time.

The Effect

The chest and shoulder muscles are the focal points of this exercise. For running as well as for balance this muscle group should not be left out in any training, since it is fundamental to free breathing.

3 Quality Stars

• Keep both arms stretched and relax your back.
• Vary the stretch by changing the distance between the hands and by slightly turning the upper body to the left and right in order to increasingly stretch the sides of the chest.

• Do this exercise with your legs together and then with your legs spread. This way, different parts of the leg muscles are affected.

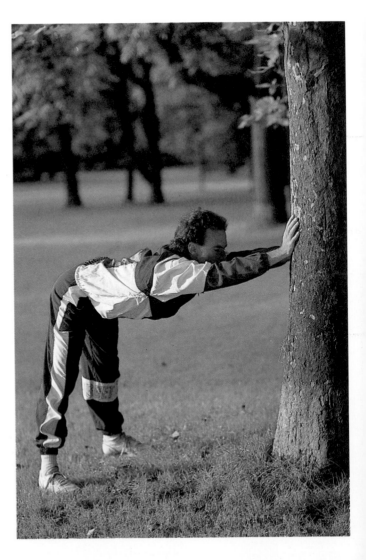

EXERCISE 3

In a standing position, prop both hands against a tree. Your legs should be in a slight stride position, and the tips of your toes should point straight ahead. Now shift your weight onto your rear leg and press your heel slowly to the floor. Remain in this position for 20 seconds and then switch legs.

The Effect

The muscular system of the calves and the Achilles tendons are stretched in this exercise. This zone is exposed to high stress with each step when running, particularly among beginners for whom irritations of the sinew can easily slow down the initial enthusiasm.

3 Quality Stars

• Intensify the exercise by setting the rear leg increasingly further back. But the heel should remain on the floor.
• The tension of the stretch can also be varied by pushing your hip forward.
• Do the points of your feet point forward? Is your extended leg stretched, so that the tension is felt all the way up to the hollow of your knee? You can easily change this exercise by bending your rear leg, so that the knee pulls forward. This way the stretch increasingly shifts to the lower calf area.

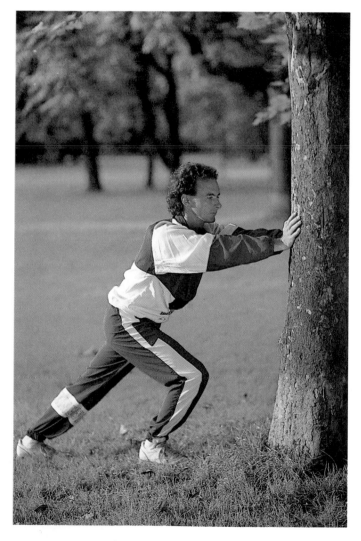

EXERCISE 4

Spread your legs slightly and
stand sideways next to the tree.
Then bend your upper body to
the side, placing both hands onto
the tree in a vertical position one
above the other, and hold this
position. Switch sides.

The Effect

The stretch affects the side of the
body and stretches the lateral stomach muscles as well as the chest
muscles.

3 Quality Stars

- In order to reach the proposed
effect, it is important that the upper body does not curl forward. Try
to take the upper shoulder back so
far that you can look up at the sky
underneath your arm. Do you feel
the difference?

- While bending to the side, pull
your left hip forward and keep both
legs stretched. That also intensifies
the stretch considerably.
- Try to bend the outer leg.

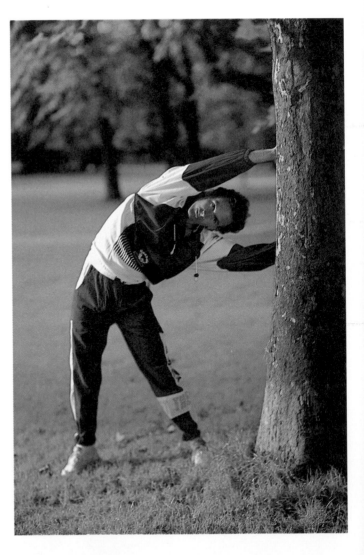

EXERCISE 5

Hang with both hands from a branch that you can easily reach, take your head back a little bit, and form a wide arch with your body.

The Effect

This is a soothing exercise, and not only after you have been running, because it offers optimal relaxation and relief for the spine and especially for the cartilage. It stretches the entire muscular system of the arms, trunk, and legs as well. Why don't you do this exercise when you go for your next walk?

3 Quality Stars

• Pick a tree with a branch that is thin enough that you can easily grasp it with your hands and low enough that you can still stand on the ground with both feet. This way you have more possibilities for bending your body in various stretches.
• Hang completely relaxed from the shoulders.
• Vary the stretch by slowly rotating the pelvis. Do you feel how the stretch wanders through various muscle regions?

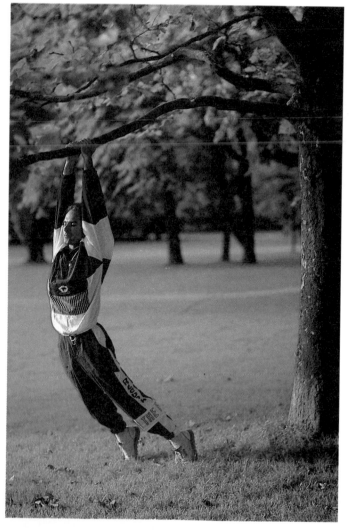

4 THE EXTRA PROGRAM TO "REFUEL"

5 Exercises to Cheer Up Drivers

Feeling "out of gas"?

You have been sitting in a car for two hours and, slowly but surely, fatigue has crept up—neck and nape become stiff, reaction-time increases, your eyes get tired, and your concentration diminishes noticeably. But you still have a long way to go. It's time for you to pep up with exercise. Therefore, stop at the next recreation area and "fuel up" with the following short exercise program.

Or have you reached your destination after a drive that seemed never-ending and tasks are waiting for you for which you have to be fresh? But you feel literally "driven-out"? This is also a moment when the extra program becomes useful.

Where does the fatigue actually come from if one has not really "done" anything? Although it may sound strange, that's just the reason—the *long, motionless sitting* is what makes you so tired. The longer the drive is, the more the natural need to move is blocked up. In addition, the seat belt has a negative effect concerning this. The muscles must be moved.

Add to this that, when driving, the breathing is limited, a lot more than when doing something more active.

This way, in the course of time, the blood supply to the muscles and brain worsens. The results are fatigue, headaches, and, in this situation, dangerous concentration weaknesses.

And then there is the *psychic* stress, caused by heavy traffic, high speed, and the need for constant attention on all sides at the same time. Through this inner tension, the muscles cramp in the nape and shoulder area particularly.

The Extra Program Is Tailored for Such Situations

- because it stimulates the breathing and blood circulation,
- because it loosens arms, shoulder girdle and nape muscles,
- because it loosens leg and back muscles,
- because it works in an altogether relaxing manner through its gentle execution and because it reduces driver stress.

All this is of distinct importance if you want to be refreshed and have good concentration for the rest of your drive after the break or if you want to loosen and relax yourself after a drive in order to be fit for new demands.

Park your car in a corner of the parking lot where you are as undisturbed as possible, and take ten minutes out of your time for the five exercises.

EXERCISE 1

Turn your back to the car and reach with both hands for the metal trim above the car doors at about 1 meter's (2½ feet's) distance. Your palms should face down. Stretch both arms and at the same time keep your upper body and your head erect and push them slightly forward. Hold this position, slowly release it, and repeat several times.

The Effect

The exercise loosens and stretches the chest and the muscular system of the lungs. Thus one can breathe deeper and freer afterwards and your entire system can be better provided with oxygen. Also, this exercise loosens your shoulder girdle and releases the tensions caused by stress.

3 Quality Stars

• Find the position that is right for your height. If the top of the car is too high, you can also try the hood and if the top seems too low, then spread your legs a bit.

• The exercise becomes more difficult the closer you push your arms together. But continue to keep your head and upper body erect; otherwise the described effect gets lost. Also try to bend the knees slightly. Do you feel the difference?

• For a change, you can push the left shoulder forward so the left side of the shoulder gets more of a "workout." Then try the right one. Try what is good for you.

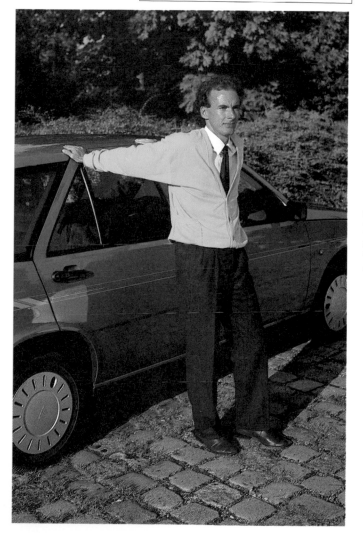

EXERCISE 2

Position yourself in front or behind the car and place the heel of your left foot onto the bumper; the standing leg remains stretched. Now bend the upper body forward from the hip joint and grasp your left upper thigh with both hands. Hold the position and switch legs.

The Effect

With this exercise you can stretch the back part of the leg muscles and activate them after they have been "paralyzed" from sitting too long. Besides this, the back muscles are mobilized as well.

3 Quality Stars

• Under no circumstance should you overstrain yourself. Hold the forward position only as long as it is comfortable for you.

• It is important that the bend forward of the upper thigh is induced from the hip area. In other words, the belly button first pulls down in the direction of the upper thigh; only then should the chest follow. The head moves forward to the ankle joint, not down to the knee.

• Are both knees still extended?

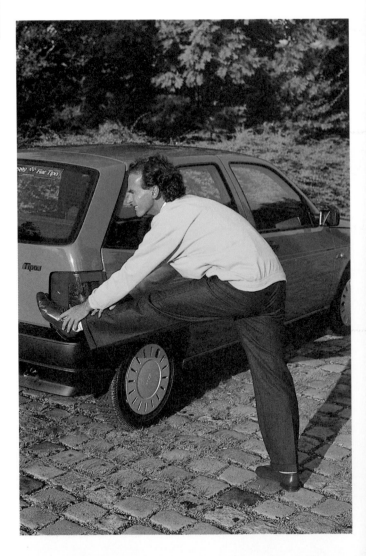

EXERCISE 3

Place the right foot on the bumper or on the tire of your car. Turn your upper body and right hip a bit to the left, so that the upper body is really positioned frontally. The tips of your toes should point away from each other. Your right hand should be propped on the right knee. The hips pull forward and down. Hold the position and switch legs.

The Effect

The inner upper-thigh muscles are the focus of this exercise. As in Exercise 2, it gives you a chance to see that your legs, after sitting for a long time, are freshly supplied with blood and are loosened up.

3 Quality Stars

• Vary the distance of the rear, stretched leg a bit, if you want the stretch to become stronger, or if the stretch becomes uncomfortable.

• In order to really concentrate the emphasis on the inner side of the muscles, it is important that your upper body is kept upright and that your hip is forward. At the same time, you can push your right knee back with your right hand.

• Try the same exercise on a bench, trash can or something similar—the main thing is that it be a bit higher.

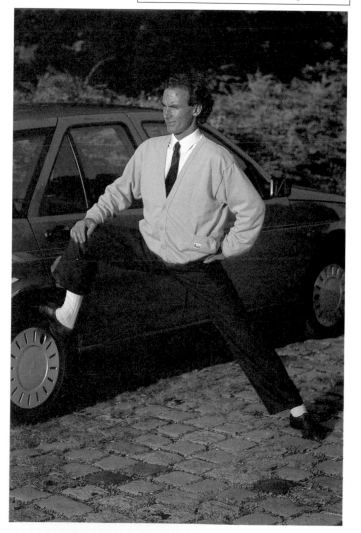

EXERCISE 4

Stand one arm's length away from the car, and prop your right hand on the car. Bend your left knee back into an angle and hold your left foot with your left hand. With your hand, pull your left foot up to your posterior and at the same time relax the left upper hand. Hold the position, then switch sides.

The Effect

The front part of the muscular system of the upper thighs and hips is stretched. After sitting for a long time, the strong bending muscles in the hip and groin area need balanced stretching in order to keep them from permanently shortening.

3 Quality Stars

• This exercise only makes sense when you are standing safely, without having to constantly balance yourself. Otherwise, the muscles get tense, and that works against a stretch that makes sense.

• The knee of the angled upper thigh should not pull sideways and down, but should remain close to the standing leg, because this way the direction of the stretch really reaches the straight upper-thigh muscles.
• Also try to grasp the bent right foot with the other hand—this way the pull of the stretch gets slightly varied.

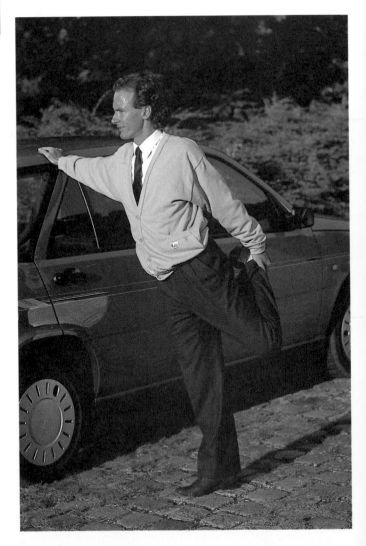

EXERCISE 5

Stand one arm's length away at the side of the car, with your legs in a stride position. The front, right leg should be bent. The right hand should be placed on the car so that the fingertips point backwards and the arm is stretched. Now turn your upper body and your head to the left, until you feel a stretch in your right shoulder. Switch sides.

The Effect

Besides the muscular system of the arms and shoulders, the muscular system of the neck is also stretched by turning the head. This improves the blood supply to the entire head area and contributes to your regaining your concentration. Even headaches that are caused by tensions in the shoulder and neck area can be soothed this way.

3 Quality Stars

• Go slowly and gently into this stretch position, because the neck and nape area are very sensitive to overstretching. This is also true for the moment when releasing the stretch.

• Pull the right shoulder forward and, at the same time, push the left shoulder backward. That way, you enhance the twist of the shoulder girdle and with that, of course, the stretch. Also, if you concentrate more on turning your upper body, you can intensify the stretch. Do not hesitate to experiment a little in order to find the optimal stretch for yourself.

• In order to reach various parts of the muscular system of the shoulders with the stretch, the right hand can be placed in different heights on the car. Do you feel how the stretch "wanders"?

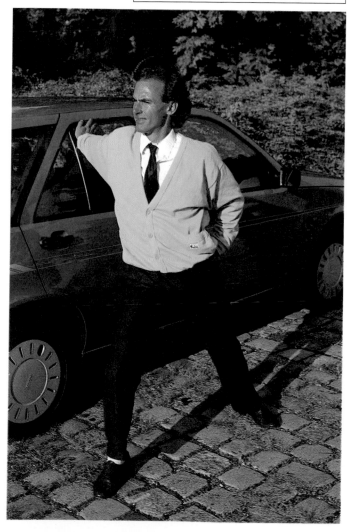

INDEX